High-Yield™

Embryology

3rd EDITION

High-Yield™
Embryology
3rd EDITION

Ronald W. Dudek, Ph.D.

Department of Anatomy and Cell Biology
Brody School of Medicine
East Carolina University
Greenville, North Carolina

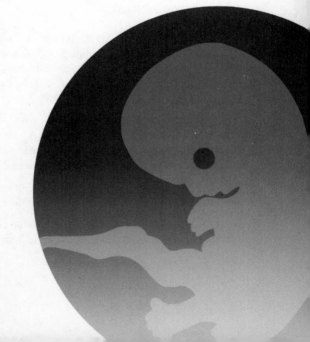

Lippincott Williams & Wilkins
a Wolters Kluwer business
Philadelphia · Baltimore · New York · London
Buenos Aires · Hong Kong · Sydney · Tokyo

Acquisitions Editor: Crystal Taylor
Managing Editor: Grace R. Caputo
Marketing Manager: Emilie Linkins
Production Editor: Sirkka E. H. Bertling
Designer: Terry Mallon
Compositor: Nesbitt Graphics, Inc.
Printer: Data Reproductions Corporation

351 West Camden Street
Baltimore, MD 21201

530 Walnut Street
Philadelphia, PA 19106

Printed in the United States of America

First Edition, 1996
Second Edition, 2001

Library of Congress Cataloging-in-Publication Data

Dudek, Ronald W., 1950-
  High-yield embryology / Ronald W. Dudek.-- 3rd ed.
      p. ; cm.
  Includes index.
  ISBN-13: 978-0-7817-6872-6
  ISBN-10: 0-7817-6872-1
  1. Embryology, Human--Outlines, syllabi, etc. I. Title.
  [DNLM: 1. Embryology--Examination Questions. 2. Embryology--Outlines. 3. Embryonic
Development--Examination Questions. 4. Embryonic Development--Outlines. 5. Fetal
Development--Examination Questions. 6. Fetal Development--Outlines. QS 618.2 D845h 2007]
QM601.D83 2007
 612.6'4--dc22

                                                             2006004275

07 08 09 10
2 3 4 5 6 7 8 9 10

Dedication

I would like to dedicate this book to my father, Stanley J. Dudek, who died Sunday, March 20, 1988, at 11 A.M. It was his hard work and sacrifice that allowed me access to the finest educational institutions in the country (St. John's University in Collegeville, MN; the University of Minnesota Medical School; Northwestern University; and the University of Chicago). It was by hard work and sacrifice that he showed his love for his wife, Lottie; daughter, Christine; and grandchildren, Karolyn, Katie, and Jeannie. I remember my father often as a good man who did the best he could. Who could ask for more? My father is missed and remembered by many.

Preface

The third edition of *High-Yield™ Embryology* marks a milestone for this book. Over the years, my didactic and organizational efforts in the first and second editions have been supplemented by the suggestions and comments from the many medical students who have used this book in preparation for the USMLE Step 1. As you may know, I include my e-mail address in the prefaces of all my books and ask for feedback from my readers. I pay close attention to these suggestions, and most have been included in this third edition. So this third edition is beautifully concise, filled with high-yield information, and presented so that its study will be highly efficient. What more could one want?

In addition, I have included a number of clinical vignettes. All these cases were written by Shawn McGill, a third-year medical student at the Brody School of Medicine. He did a wonderful job with these, including quotations from the patients or the patients' parents of the sort that you will often hear in the clinic.

I would appreciate receiving your comments or suggestions concerning *High-Yield™ Embryology*, 3rd edition, especially after you have taken the USMLE Step 1. Your suggestions will find their way into the fourth edition. You may contact me at dudekr@ecu.edu.

Contents

Chapter 1

Prefertilization Events

I **Gametes** (oocytes and spermatozoa), descendants of **primordial germ cells,** are produced in the adult by either **oogenesis** or **spermatogenesis,** processes that involve **meiosis.** Primordial germ cells originate in the **wall of the yolk sac** of the embryo and migrate into the gonadal region.

II **Meiosis (Figure 1-1),** which occurs **only during the production of gametes,** consists of two cell divisions **(meiosis I and meiosis II)** and results in the formation of gametes containing 23 chromosomes and 1N amount of DNA **(23,1N).** Meiosis:

  A. Reduces the number of chromosomes within the gametes to ensure that the number of chromosomes (46) for the human species is maintained from generation to generation.
  B. Redistributes maternal and paternal chromosomes to ensure genetic variability.
  C. Promotes the exchange of small amounts of maternal and paternal DNA via **crossover** during meiosis I.

III **Female Gametogenesis (Oogenesis)**

  A. **Primordial germ cells (46,2N)** from the wall of the yolk sac arrive in the ovary at week 4 of embryonic development and differentiate into **oogonia (46,2N).**
  B. Oogonia enter **meiosis I** and undergo DNA replication to form **primary oocytes (46,4N).** All primary oocytes are formed by the **fifth month of fetal life** and remain dormant in **prophase (diplotene) of meiosis I until puberty.**
  C. During a woman's ovarian cycle, a primary oocyte completes meiosis I to form a **secondary oocyte (23,2N)** and a **first polar body,** which probably degenerates.
  D. The secondary oocyte enters **meiosis II,** and ovulation occurs when the chromosomes align at metaphase. The secondary oocyte remains **arrested in metaphase of meiosis II** until fertilization occurs.
  E. At fertilization, the secondary oocyte completes meiosis II to form a **mature oocyte (23,1N)** and a **second polar body.**

IV **Hormonal Control of the Female Reproductive Cycle (Figure 1-2)**

  A. The hypothalamus secretes **gonadotropin-releasing hormone (Gn-RH).**
  B. In response to GnRH, the adenohypophysis secretes the gonadotropins, **follicle-stimulating hormone (FSH),** and **luteinizing hormone (LH).**
  C. FSH stimulates the development of a secondary follicle into a Graafian follicle within the ovary.
  D. Granulosa cells of the secondary and Graafian follicle secrete **estrogen (E).**
  E. E stimulates the endometrium of the uterus to enter the proliferative phase.
  F. LH stimulates ovulation.
  G. Following ovulation, granulosa lutein cells of the corpus luteum secrete **progesterone (P).**
  H. P stimulates the endometrium of the uterus to enter the secretory phase.

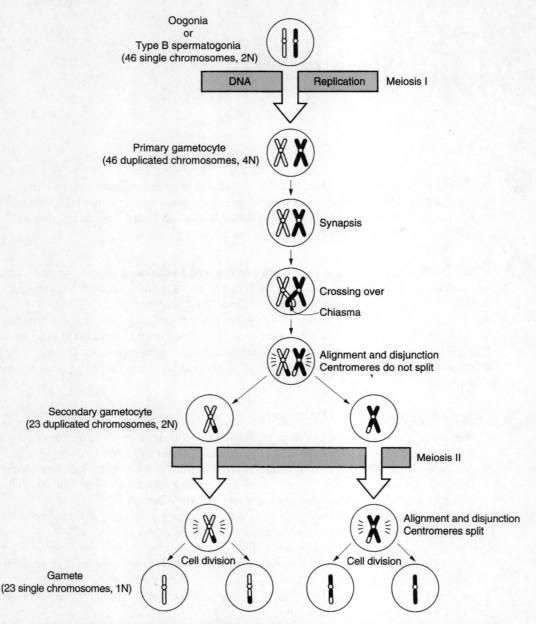

NUMBER OF CHROMOSOMES AND AMOUNT OF DNA CONTAINED IN CELLS DURING THE STAGE OF GAMETOGENESIS

Cell Type	Number of Chromosomes, Amount of DNA
Primordial germ cell, oogonia, spermatogonia (types A and B), zygote, blastomeres, all normal somatic cells	46,2N
Primary oocyte, primary spermatocyte	46,4N
Secondary oocyte, secondary spermatocyte	23,2N
Oocyte (ovum), spermatid, sperm	23,1N

● **Figure 1.1 Meiosis.** This schematic representation of meiosis I and meiosis II emphasizes the chromosomal changes and amount of DNA that occur during either oogenesis or spermatogenesis. Note that only one pair of homologous chromosomes is shown (white = maternal origin and black = paternal origin). Synapsis is the pairing of homologous chromosomes. The point at which the DNA molecule crosses over is called the chiasma; this is where exchange of small amounts of maternal and paternal DNA occurs. Note that synapsis and crossing over occur only during meiosis I.

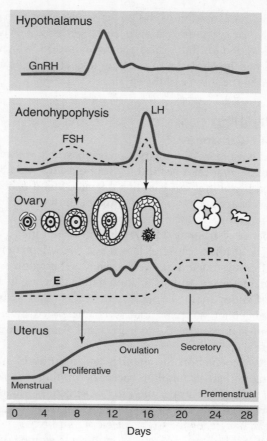

● **Figure 1.2 Hormonal control of the female reproductive cycle.** The various patterns of hormone secretion from the hypothalamus, adenohypophysis, and ovary are shown. These hormones prepare the endometrium of the uterus for implantation of a conceptus. The menstrual cycle of the uterus includes the following: (1) the **menstrual phase** (days 1–4), characterized by the **necrosis and shedding** of the functional layer of the endometrium; (2) the **proliferative phase** (days 4–15), characterized by the **regeneration** of the functional layer of the endometrium and a **low basal body temperature** (97.5°F); (3) the **ovulatory phase** (days 14–16), characterized by **ovulation** of a secondary oocyte and coincides with the LH surge; (4) the **secretory phase** (days 15–25), characterized by **secretory activity** of the endometrial glands and an **elevated basal body temperature** (over 98°F)—this is the phase during which implantation of the conceptus occurs; and (5) the premenstrual phase (days 25–28), characterized by **ischemia** due to reduced blood flow to the endometrium.

 Male Gametogenesis (Spermatogenesis) is classically divided into three phases: spermatocytogenesis, meiosis, and spermiogenesis.

A. Spermatocytogenesis. Primordial germ cells (46,2N) from the wall of the yolk sac arrive in the testes at week 4 of embryonic development and remain dormant until puberty. At puberty, primordial germ cells differentiate into **type A spermatogonia (46,2N).** Type A spermatogonia undergo **mitosis** to provide a continuous supply of stem cells throughout the reproductive life of the male (a process called spermatocytogenesis). Some type A spermatogonia differentiate into **type B spermatogonia (46,2N).**

B. Meiosis. Type B spermatogonia enter meiosis I and undergo DNA replication to form **primary spermatocytes (46,4N).** Primary spermatocytes complete meiosis I to form two **secondary spermatocytes (23,2N).** Secondary spermatocytes complete meiosis II to form four **spermatids (23,1N).**

C. Spermiogenesis. Spermatids undergo a **postmeiotic series of morphological changes** (called spermiogenesis) to form **sperm (23,1N).** These changes include formation of the acrosome, condensation of the nucleus, and formation of the head, neck, and tail. The total time for sperm formation is about 64 days. Newly ejaculated sperm are incapable of fertilization until they undergo **capacitation,** which occurs in the female reproductive tract and involves the unmasking of sperm glycosyltransferases and removal of proteins coating the surface of the sperm.

VI Clinical Correlations

A. **Offspring of older women**
   1. Prolonged dormancy of primary oocytes may be the reason for the high incidence of chromosomal abnormalities in offspring of older women. Since all primary oocytes are formed by month 5 of fetal life, a female infant is born with her entire supply of gametes. Primary oocytes remain dormant until ovulation; those ovulated late in the woman's reproductive life may have been dormant for as long as 40 years.
   2. The incidence of **trisomy 21 (Down syndrome)** increases with advanced age of the mother. The primary cause of Down syndrome is maternal meiotic nondisjunction. Clinical findings include: severe mental retardation, epicanthal folds, Brushfield spots, simian creases, and association with a decrease in alpha fetoprotein.
B. **Offspring of older men.** An increased incidence of **achondroplasia** (an autosomal dominant congenital skeletal anomaly characterized by retarded bone growth in the limbs with normal-sized head and trunk) and **Marfan syndrome** is associated with advanced paternal age.
C. **Male fertility** depends on the number and motility of sperm. Fertile males produce from 20 to more than 100 million sperm per milliliter of semen. Sterile males produce less than 10 million sperm per milliliter of semen. Normally up to 10% of sperm in an ejaculate may be grossly deformed (two heads or two tails); but these sperm probably do not fertilize an oocyte, owing to their lack of motility.
D. **Anovulation** is the absence of ovulation in some women due to inadequate secretion of FSH and LH, which is often treated with **clomiphene citrate** (a fertility drug). Clomiphene citrate competes with estrogen for binding sites in the adenohypophysis, thereby suppressing the normal negative feedback loop of estrogen on the adenohypophysis. This stimulates FSH and LH secretion and induces ovulation.
E. **Hormonal contraception**
   1. **Oral contraceptives**
      a. **Combination pills** contain a combination of **estrogen and progesterone.** They are taken for 21 days and then discontinued for 7 days. The primary mechanism of action is the inhibition of GnRH, FSH, and LH secretion, thereby preventing ovulation.
      b. **Progesterone-only pills** contain only **progesterone.** They are taken continuously without a break. The primary mechanism of action is not known, but thickening of the cervical mucus (hostile to sperm migration) and thinning of the endometrium (leaving it unprepared for the implantation of a conceptus) are known to occur.
   2. **Medroxyprogesterone acetate (Depo-Provera)** is a progesterone-only product that offers a long-acting alternative to oral contraceptives. It can be injected **intramuscularly** and will prevent ovulation **for 2–3 months.**
   3. **Levonorgestrel (Norplant)** is a progesterone-only product that offers an even longer-acting alternative to oral contraceptives. The capsules containing levonorgestrel can be implanted **subdermally** and will prevent ovulation for **1–5 years.**
   4. **Seasonale** is a product that combines ethinyl estradiol (0.03 mg) and levonorgestrel (0.15 mg); it is an **extended-cycle** oral contraceptive. Seasonale has a 91-day treatment cycle whereby the woman may expect to have only four menstrual periods per year.
   5. **Ortho Evra** is a product combining ethinyl estradiol (0.75 mg) and norelgestromin (6.0 mg); it is delivered by a transdermal patch.

6. **Emergency contraceptive pills (ECPs) or postcoital contraception.** ECPs are sometimes called **"morning-after pills,"** but the pills can be started right away or up to 5 days after the woman has had unprotected sex. This therapy is more effective the earlier it is initiated within a **120-hour window.** There are two types of ECPs:

   a. **Combined ECPs** contain both estrogen and progesterone in the same dosage as ordinary birth control pills. In many countries (but not the United States), combined ECPs are specially packaged and labeled for emergency use. However, not all brands of birth control pills can be used for emergency contraception (for more information, see www.not-2-late.com). The dosage of **Ogestrel** and **Ovral** is 2 pills within 120 hours after unprotected sex followed by 2 more pills 12 hours later. Combined ECPs are associated with a high incidence of nausea and vomiting.

   b. **Progesterone-only ECPs** contain only **progesterone.** The brand name in the United States is **Plan B** (0.75 mg levonorgestrel). The dosage of Plan B is 1 pill within 72 hours of unprotected sex; the second pill is to be taken 12 hours after the first pill. Plan B is associated with a reduced incidence of nausea and vomiting.

   c. **Diethylstilbestrol (DES)** was used as an ECP in the past but has been discontinued, since it is associated with reproductive tract anomalies and vaginal cancers in exposed offspring. **Clear cell adenocarcinoma of the vagina** occurs in daughters of women who were exposed to DES therapy during pregnancy. A precursor to clear cell adenocarcinoma is **vaginal adenosis** (a benign condition), where stratified squamous epithelium is replaced by mucosal columnar epithelium-lined crypts.

7. **Luteinizing hormone–releasing hormone (LH–RH) analogues.** Chronic treatment with an LH–RH analogue (e.g., **buserelin**) paradoxically results in the down-regulation of FSH and LH secretion, thereby preventing ovulation.

Chapter 2

Week 1 (Days 1–7)*

I **Overview.** Figure 2-1 summarizes the events that occur during week 1, following fertilization.

II **Fertilization** occurs in the **ampulla of the uterine tube.**
  A. The sperm binds to the zona pellucida of the secondary oocyte, arrested in metaphase of meiosis II, and triggers the **acrosome reaction,** causing the release of acrosomal enzymes (e.g., **acrosin**).
  B. Aided by the acrosomal enzymes, the sperm penetrates the zona pellucida. Penetration of the zona pellucida elicits the **cortical reaction,** rendering the secondary oocyte **impermeable to other sperm.**
  C. The sperm and secondary oocyte cell membranes fuse, and the contents of the sperm enter the cytoplasm of the oocyte. The male genetic material forms the **male pronucleus.** The tail and mitochondria of the sperm degenerate. Therefore all mitochondria within the zygote are of maternal origin (i.e., **all mitochondrial DNA is of maternal origin**).
  D. The secondary oocyte completes meiosis II, forming a mature **ovum.** The nucleus of the ovum is the **female pronucleus.**
  E. The male and female pronuclei fuse to form a **zygote.**

III **Cleavage** is a series of **mitotic** divisions of the zygote. The zygote cytoplasm is successively cleaved to form a **blastula,** consisting of increasingly smaller **blastomeres** (e.g., the first blastomere stage consists of 2 cells; the next, 4 cells; the next, 8 cells, and so on). At the 16- to 32-cell stage, the blastomeres form a **morula,** consisting of an **inner cell mass** and **outer cell mass.** Blastomeres are considered **totipotent** up to the 8-cell stage (i.e., each blastomere can form a complete embryo by itself, which is important in considering monozygotic twinning).

IV **Blastocyst Formation** occurs when fluid secreted within the morula forms the **blastocyst cavity.** The inner cell mass, which becomes the **embryo,** is now called the **embryoblast.** The outer cell mass, which becomes part of the **placenta,** is now called the **trophoblast.**

V **Implantation.** The **zona pellucida must degenerate** for implantation to occur. The blastocyst implants within the **posterosuperior wall** of the uterus. The blastocyst implants within the **functional layer of the endometrium** during the **secretory phase** of the menstrual cycle. The trophoblast differentiates into the **cytotrophoblast** and **syncytiotrophoblast.**

---

*The age of the developing conceptus can be measured either from the estimated day of fertilization (**fertilization age**) or from the day of the last normal menstrual period (**LNMP**). In this book, ages are presented as fertilization age.

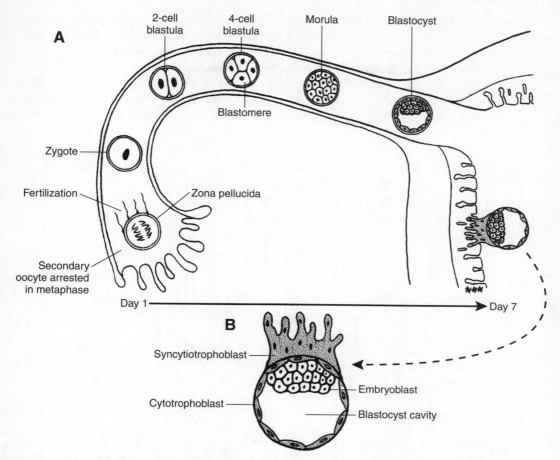

 Figure 2.1 The stages of human development. (A) The stages of human development during week 1. **(B)** A day 7 blastocyst.

VI Clinical Correlations

A. Ectopic tubal pregnancy (ETP)

1. An ETP occurs when the blastocyst implants within the uterine tube due to **delayed transport.** The **ampulla of the uterine tube** is the most common site of an ETP. The **rectouterine pouch (pouch of Douglas)** is a common site for an ectopic abdominal pregnancy.

2. **Chronic salpingitis, endometriosis,** and **postoperative adhesions are** frequently predisposing conditions for an ETP.

3. An ETP is most commonly seen in women with **endometriosis** or **pelvic inflammatory disease.**

4. An ETP leads to uterine tube rupture and hemorrhage if surgical intervention (i.e., salpingectomy) is not performed.

5. An ETP presents with **abnormal uterine bleeding, unilateral pelvic pain, increased levels of HCG** (but lower than originally expected with a uterine implantation pregnancy), and a **massive first-trimester bleed.**

6. An ETP must be differentially diagnosed from **appendicitis,** an **aborting intrauterine pregnancy,** or a **bleeding corpus luteum** of a normal intrauterine pregnancy.

B. Twinning (Figure 2-2)

1. **Dizygotic (fraternal) twins** result from the fertilization of two different secondary oocytes by two different sperm; the resulting two zygotes form two blastocysts, each

of which implants separately into the endometrium of the uterus. Hence the twins are no more genetically alike than siblings born at different times. Dizygotic twins and 35% of monozygotic twins have **two placentas, two amniotic sacs**, and **two chorions (i.e., a diamnionic-dichorionic membrane).**

2. **Monozygotic (identical) twins** result from the fertilization of one secondary oocyte by one sperm. The resulting zygote forms a blastocyst in which the inner cell mass (embryoblast) splits into two. Hence, the twins are genetically identical. In 65% of

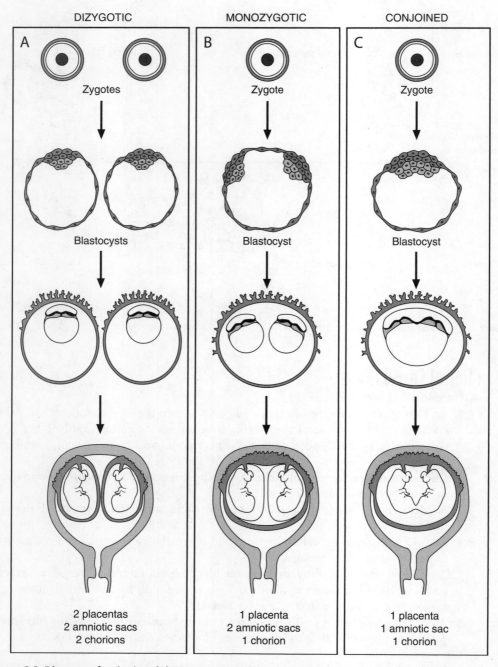

DIZYGOTIC	MONOZYGOTIC	CONJOINED
A	B	C
Zygotes	Zygote	Zygote
Blastocysts	Blastocyst	Blastocyst
2 placentas 2 amniotic sacs 2 chorions	1 placenta 2 amniotic sacs 1 chorion	1 placenta 1 amniotic sac 1 chorion

● **Figure 2.2 Diagram of twinning. (A)** Dizygotic twins. **(B)** Monozygotic twins. **(C)** Conjoined twins.

the cases, monozygotic twins have **one placenta, two amniotic sacs**, and **one chorion (i.e., a diamnionic-monochorionic membrane).**

3. Conjoined (Siamese) twins form exactly like monozygotic twins except that the inner cell mass (embryoblast) does not completely split. Hence two embryos form, but they are joined by tissue bridges at various regions of the body (e.g., head, thorax, or pelvis).

C. In vitro fertilization (Figure 2-3) requires the sequential application of a number of techniques, as indicated below.

1. Clomiphene citrate is administered to stimulate multiple ovulation.

2. Oocytes are collected by needle aspiration from the ovary, assisted by ultrasound visualization.

3. Sperm are collected by masturbation; the sperm are separated from seminal fluid and undergo capacitation by exposure to ionic solutions. In cases of oligospermia (infertility due to a low sperm count), multiple samples may be obtained over an extended period of time.

4. Sperm and oocytes are cultured together. The success of in vitro fertilization is judged by the presence of two pronuclei with the oocyte.

5. Cleavage is allowed to proceed in vitro to the eight-cell-stage embryo.

6. Typically, at least three embryos are transferred to the uterus, because implantation has a low success rate.

7. If the first embryo transfer does not result in a pregnancy, the remaining embryos are frozen for future use.

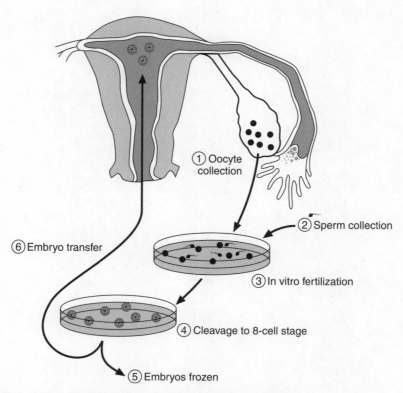

● **Figure 2.3 Diagram of various steps involved in in vitro fertilization.**

Case Study

A 25-year-old woman comes into your office complaining of "spotting" and "stomach pains" as she points to her lower abdomen. She notes that she and her husband have been trying to initiate a pregnancy and that she had her last period about 5 weeks earlier. She says that after talking with her girlfriends about her symptoms, she became worried about what it could be, so she decided to pay you a visit. Her chart shows that she has a history of pelvic inflammatory disease. What is the most likely diagnosis?

Differentials

- Ectopic pregnancy, spontaneous abortion, pelvic inflammatory disease

Relevant Physical Exam Findings

- A tender pelvic mass is palpable.
- There is amenorrhea.
- Light vaginal bleeding is noted.
- The patient has lower abdominal pain.

Relevant Lab Findings

- Elevated β-hCG but lower than expected for pregnancy
- Lower than normal progesterone
- Absence of intrauterine pregnancy on ultrasound. However, implantation in the ampulla of the left uterine tube is detected.

Diagnosis

- Ectopic pregnancy

Chapter 3

Week 2 (Days 8–14)

I **Embryoblast** **(Figure 3-1).** The embryoblast differentiates into two distinct cell layers: the dorsal **epiblast** and the ventral **hypoblast.** The epiblast and hypoblast together form a flat, ovoid disk known as the **bilaminar embryonic disk.**

A. Within the epiblast, clefts develop and eventually coalesce to form the **amniotic cavity.**

B. Hypoblast cells migrate and line the inner surface of the cytotrophoblast, eventually delimiting a space called the definitive **yolk sac.**

C. The epiblast and hypoblast fuse to form the **prochordal plate,** which marks the future site of the **mouth.**

II **Trophoblast**

A. The syncytiotrophoblast continues its growth into the endometrium to make contact with endometrial blood vessels and glands. The syncytiotrophoblast **does not divide mitotically.** It produces **human chorionic gonadotropin (hCG).**

B. The cytotrophoblast does divide mitotically, adding to the growth of the syncytiotrophoblast. **Primary chorionic villi** formed by the cytotrophoblast protrude into the syncytiotrophoblast.

III **Extraembryonic Mesoderm** is a new layer of cells derived from the epiblast.

A. **Extraembryonic somatic mesoderm (somatopleuric mesoderm)** lines the cytotrophoblast, forms the **connecting stalk,** and covers the amnion (see Figure 3-1). The conceptus is suspended by the connecting stalk within the **chorionic cavity.** The wall of the chorionic cavity is called the **chorion** and consists of three components: **extraembryonic somatic mesoderm, cytotrophoblast,** and **syncytiotrophoblast.**

B. **Extraembryonic visceral mesoderm (splanchnopleuric mesoderm)** covers the yolk sac.

IV **Clinical Correlations**

A. **Human chorionic gonadotropin (hCG)** is a glycoprotein produced by the syncytiotrophoblasts, which stimulates the production of progesterone by the corpus luteum of the ovary (i.e., it maintains corpus luteum function). This is clinically significant, since progesterone produced by the corpus luteum is essential for the maintenance of pregnancy until week 8. The placenta then takes over progesterone production. hCG can be assayed in **maternal blood at day 8** or **maternal urine at day 10** and is the basis of pregnancy testing. hCG is detectable throughout a pregnancy. **Low hCG values** may predict a spontaneous abortion or indicate an ectopic pregnancy. **Elevated hCG values** may indicate a multiple pregnancy, hydatidiform mole, or gestational trophoblastic neoplasia (such as choriocarcinoma).

B. **RU-486 (mifepristone; Mifeprex)** will initiate menstruation when taken within 8–10 weeks of the start of the last menstrual period. If implantation of a conceptus has occurred, the conceptus will be sloughed along with the endometrium. RU-486 is a

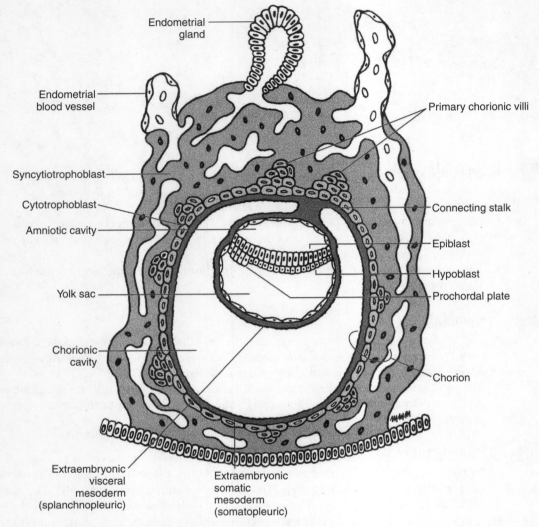

Endometrial gland

Endometrial blood vessel

Primary chorionic villi

Syncytiotrophoblast

Cytotrophoblast

Connecting stalk

Amniotic cavity

Epiblast

Hypoblast

Yolk sac

Prochordal plate

Chorionic cavity

Chorion

Extraembryonic visceral mesoderm (splanchnopleuric)

Extraembryonic somatic mesoderm (somatopleuric)

● **Figure 3.1 Day-14 blastocyst.** A day-14 blastocyst highlighting the formation of the bilaminar embryonic disk and the completion of implantation within the endometrium.

progesterone receptor antagonist (blocker) used in conjunction with misoprostol (Cytotec; an analogue of prostaglandin E_1, or PGE_1) and is 96% effective at terminating a pregnancy.

C. **Hydatidiform mole (complete or partial; Figure 3-2A,B).** A blighted blastocyst (i.e., blastocyst growth is prevented) leads to death of the embryo. This is followed by hyperplastic proliferation of the trophoblast. A hydatidiform mole (complete or partial) represents an abnormal placenta characterized by marked enlargement of chorionic villi. A complete mole (no embryo present) is distinguished from a partial mole (embryo present) by the amount of chorionic villous involvement. The hallmarks of a complete mole include gross, generalized edema of chorionic villi, forming grape-like, transparent vesicles; hyperplastic proliferation of surrounding trophoblastic cells; and absence of an embryo/fetus. Clinical signs diagnostic of a mole include preeclampsia during the first trimester, elevated hCG levels (>100,000 mIU/mL), and an enlarged uterus with bleeding. Follow-up visits are essential after a mole because 3%–5% of moles develop into gestational trophoblastic neoplasia.

D. Gestational trophoblastic neoplasia (GTN, or choriocarcinoma; Figure 3-2C,D). GTN is a malignant tumor of the trophoblast that may occur following a normal or ectopic pregnancy, abortion, or hydatidiform mole. With a high degree of suspicion, elevated HCG levels are diagnostic. Nonmetastatic GTN (i.e., confined to the uterus) is the most common form of this neoplasia and treatment is highly successful. However, the prognosis of metastatic GTN is poor if it spreads to the liver or brain.

E. Oncofetal antigens (Table 3-1) are cell-surface antigens that normally appear only on embryonic cells; for unknown reasons, however, they reexpress themselves in human malignant cells. Monoclonal antibodies directed against specific oncofetal antigens provide an avenue for cancer therapy.

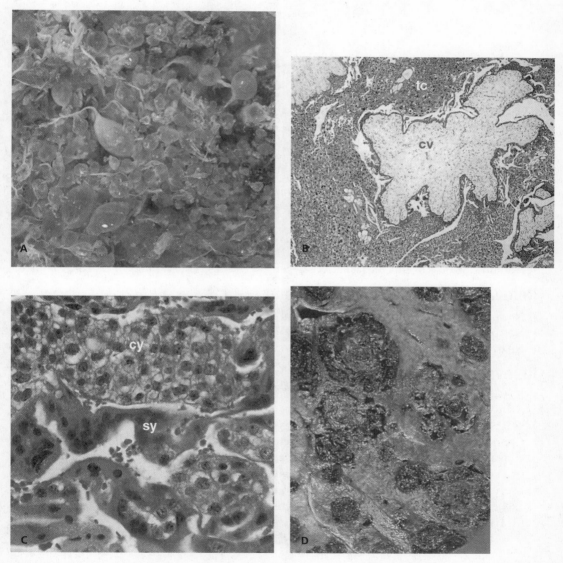

● **Figure 3.2 (A,B) Hydatidiform mole.** The photograph shows gross edema of the chorionic villi, forming grape-like vesicles. Light micrograph (LM) shows edema of the chorionic villi (cv) surrounded by hyperplastic trophoblastic cells (tc). **(C,D) Gestational trophoblastic neoplasia.** LM shows the distinctive alternating arrangement of mononuclear cytotrophoblastic cells (cy) and multinucleated syncytiotrophoblastic cells (sy). This photograph shows hemorrhagic nodules metastatic to the liver; they are due to the rapid proliferation of trophoblastic cells combined with a marked propensity to invade blood vessels. The central portion of the lesion is hemorrhagic and necrotic, with only a thin rim of trophoblastic cells at the periphery.

TABLE 3-1	ONCOFETAL ANTIGEN PANEL
Antigen	**Associated Tumor**
α-Fetoprotein	Hepatoma, germ cell neoplasms
Carcinoembryonic antigen (CEA)	Colorectal cancer, breast cancer, others
$β_2$-Microglobulin	Lymphoma
CA 125	Ovarian cancer
CA 15-3	Breast cancer
CA 19-9	Pancreatic cancer
Neuron-specific enolase	Endocrine neoplasms, small cell carcinoma, seminoma
Prostate-specific antigen (PSA)	Prostate cancer

CA = cancer antigen

Case Study

A 31-year-old woman comes into the office complaining of "running a fever," being nauseated, and losing weight—"about 15 pounds or so"—over the preceding month. She tells you that she had a miscarriage about 2 months earlier and "all of a sudden these other problems came up." She adds that the doctors said she had preeclampsia during her first trimester of this recent pregnancy. She says that she was supposed to come back in but didn't because she "felt depressed about losing the baby." She remarks that she hasn't made any changes in her diet and that she "thought she would have gained weight with all the food she was eating." What is the most likely diagnosis?

Differentials

- Malnutrition, loss of appetite, achalasia, hyperthyroidism, cachexia from a malignant tumor

Relevant Physical Exam Findings

- Normal thyroid upon palpation
- No coughing blood
- No diarrhea

Relevant Lab Findings

- Elevated hCG

Diagnosis

- Choriocarcinoma. This is a result of her premalignant condition of hydatidiform mole, which presents with preeclampsia during the first trimester and elevated hCG, progressing to a gestational trophoblastic neoplasia. Malnutrition and loss of appetite are excluded because the patient mentioned that she was eating a lot of food. Hyperthyroidism was excluded because the lab report did not mention an elevated thyroid-stimulating hormone (TSH).

Chapter 4

Embryonic Period (Weeks 3–8)

I **Introduction.** All major organ systems begin to develop during the embryonic period, causing a **craniocaudal** and **lateral body folding** of the embryo. By the end of the embryonic period (week 8), the embryo has a distinct human appearance. During the embryonic period, the basic segmentation of the human embryo in a craniocaudal direction is controlled by the ***Hox* (homeobox) complex** of genes. All Hox genes contain a sequence of 180 base pairs (**homeobox**) encoding a region (**homeodomain**) 60 amino acids long, which binds to DNA. All homeodomain proteins are gene-regulatory proteins (i.e., they control transcription).

II **Gastrulation** (Figure 4-1) is a process that establishes the three primary germ layers **(ectoderm, mesoderm, and endoderm)**, thereby forming a **trilaminar embryonic disk.** This process is first indicated by the formation of the **primitive streak** within the epiblast.
A. Ectoderm gives further rise to **neuroectoderm** and **neural crest cells.**
B. Endoderm remains intact.
C. Mesoderm gives further rise to **paraxial mesoderm** (somitomeres and 35 pairs of somites), **intermediate mesoderm,** and **lateral mesoderm.**
D. All adult cells and tissues can trace their embryological origin back to the three primary germ layers (Table 4-1).

III **Clinical Correlations**
A. A chordoma (CD) is either a benign or malignant tumor that arises from remnants of the **notochord.** A CD may be found either intracranially or in the sacral region and occurs more commonly in men late in adult life (age 50).
B. The first missed menstrual period is usually the **first indication of pregnancy.** Week 3 of embryonic development coincides with the first missed menstrual period. Note that at this time the embryo has already undergone 2 weeks of development. It is crucial that the woman become aware of her pregnancy as soon as possible because the embryonic period is a period of **high susceptibility to teratogens**.
C. A sacrococcygeal teratoma (ST; Figure 4-2A) is a tumor that arises from remnants of the **primitive streak,** which normally degenerates and disappears. The ST is derived from pluripotent cells of the primitive streak and often contains various types of tissue (e.g., bone, nerve, hair). It occurs more commonly in female infants and usually becomes malignant during infancy (must be removed by age 6 months).
D. Caudal dysplasia (sirenomelia; Figure 4-2B) comprises a constellation of syndromes ranging from minor lesions of the lower vertebrae to complete fusion of the lower limbs. Caudal dysplasia is caused by abnormal gastrulation, in which the migration of mesoderm is disturbed. It can be associated with various cranial anomalies:
 1. VATER, an acronym for **v**ertebral defects, **a**nal atresia, **t**racheo**e**sophageal fistula, and **r**enal defects.
 2. VACTERL, which is similar to VATER but also includes cardiovascular defects and upper **l**imb defects.

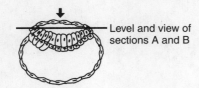

Level and view of
sections A and B

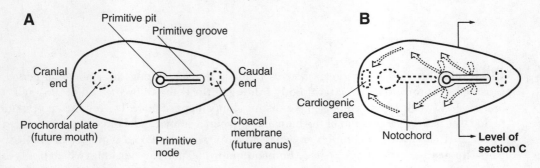

A

Primitive pit
Primitive groove

Cranial
end

Caudal
end

Prochordal plate
(future mouth)

Primitive
node

Cloacal
membrane
(future anus)

B

Cardiogenic
area

Notochord

Level of
section C

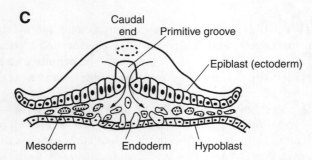

C

Caudal
end   Primitive groove

Epiblast (ectoderm)

Mesoderm   Endoderm   Hypoblast

● **Figure 4.1 Gastrulation.** The embryoblast at the upper left is provided for orientation. **(A)** Dorsal view of the epiblast. The primitive streak consists of the primitive groove, node, and pit. **(B)** Arrows show the migration of cells through the primitive streak. The notochord (i.e., mesoderm located between the primitive node and prochordal plate) induces the formation of the neural tube. The cardiogenic area is the future site of the heart. **(C)** Epiblast cells migrate to the primitive streak and insert themselves between the epiblast and hypoblast. Some epiblast cells displace the hypoblast to form endoderm; the remainder migrate cranially, laterally, and along the midline to form mesoderm. After gastrulation, the epiblast is called ectoderm.

TABLE 4-1	SUMMARY OF GERM LAYER DERIVATIVES	
Ectoderm	**Mesoderm**	**Endoderm**
Epidermis, hair, nails, sweat and sebaceous glands	Muscle (smooth, cardiac, skeletal)	Hepatocytes
Utricle, semicircular ducts, vestibular ganglion of CN VIII	Extraocular muscles, ciliary muscle of eye, iris stroma, ciliary body stroma, substantia propria of cornea, corneal endothelium, sclera, choroid	Principal and oxyphil cells of parathyroid
Saccule, cochlear duct (organ of Corti), spiral ganglion of CN VIII		Thyroid follicular cells
Olfactory placode, CN I		Epithelial reticular cells of thymus
Ameloblasts (enamel of teeth)	Muscles of tongue (occipital somites)	Acinar and islet cells of pancreas
Adenohypophysis	Pharyngeal arch muscles	Acinar cells of submandibular and sublingual glands
Lens of eye	Laryngeal cartilages	*Epithelial lining of:*
Anterior epithelium of cornea	Connective tissue	GI tract
Acinar cells of parotid gland	Dermis and subcutaneous layer of skin	Trachea, bronchi, lungs
Acinar cells of mammary gland	Bone and cartilage	Biliary apparatus
Epithelial lining of:	Dura mater	Urinary bladder, female urethra, most of male urethra
Lower anal canal	Endothelium of blood and lymph vessels	Inferior two-thirds of vagina
Distal part of male urethra	RBCs, WBCs, microglia, and Kupffer cells	Auditory tube, middle ear cavity
External auditory meatus	Spleen	Crypts of palatine tonsils
Neuroectoderm	Kidney	
All neurons within brain and spinal cord (CNS)	Adrenal cortex	
Retina, iris epithelium, ciliary body epithelium, optic nerve (CNII), optic chiasm, optic tract, dilator and sphincter pupillae muscles	Testes, epididymis, ductus deferens, seminal vesicle, ejaculatory duct	
Astrocytes, oligodendrocytes, ependymocytes, tanycytes, choroid plexus cells	Ovary, uterus, uterine tubes, superior third of vagina	
Neurohypophysis		
Pineal gland		
Neural Crest		
Neurons within ganglia (dorsal root, cranial, autonomic)		
Schwann cells		
Odontoblasts (dentin of teeth)		
Pia and arachnoid		
Chromaffin cells (adrenal medulla)		
Parafollicular (C) cells of thyroid		
Melanocytes		
Aorticopulmonary septum		
Pharyngeal arch skeletal components		
Bones of neurocranium		

CN = cranial nerve; CNS = central nervous system; GI = gastrointestinal; RBCs = red blood cells; WBCs = white blood cells.

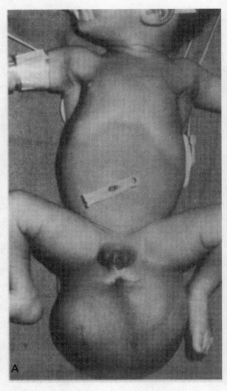 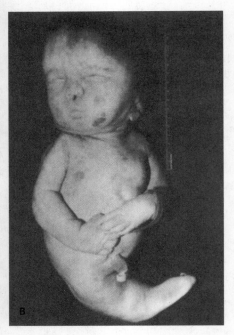

● **Figure 4.2** **(A) Infant with a sacrococcygeal teratoma. (B) Infant with caudal dysplasia (sirenomelia).**

Case Study

A distraught mother brings her 2-month-old daughter in to your office saying that she has noticed a "lump growing from the child's bottom." She "noticed it about two weeks ago while changing her diaper." It was small so she didn't think much of it, but over time it "grew to the size of a baseball." What is the most likely diagnosis?

Differentials

- Sacrococcygeal teratoma, spina bifida with meningocele, spina bifida with meningomyelocele

Relevant Physical Exam Findings

- Large spheroid mass that appears to be very firm on palpation

Relevant Lab Findings

- Biopsy of the mass shows tissue containing hair, teeth, muscle fibers, and thyroid follicular cells.

Diagnosis

- Sacrococcygeal teratoma is a remnant of the primitive streak that contains all three germ layers: ectoderm (hair and teeth), mesoderm (muscle fibers), and endoderm (thyroid follicular cells). A sacrococcygeal teratoma is different from spina bifida with meningocele or spina bifida with meningomyelocele, which stem from a failure of the bony vertebral arches to fuse with the sac containing cerebrospinal fluid.

Chapter 5

Placenta, Amniotic Fluid, and Umbilical Cord

ⓘ **Placenta** **(Figure 5-1).** The placenta, formed as the endometrium of the uterus, is invaded by the developing embryo as the trophoblast forms the villous chorion. The formation of the villous chorion goes through three stages: **primary chorionic villi, secondary chorionic villi,** and **tertiary chorionic villi.**

A. Components

1. **The maternal component** of the placenta consists of the **decidua basalis,** which is derived from the endometrium of the uterus located between the blastocyst and the myometrium. The decidua basalis and **decidua parietalis** (which includes all portions of the endometrium other than the site of implantation) are shed as part of the afterbirth. The **decidua capsularis,** the portion of endometrium that covers the blastocyst and separates it from the uterine cavity, becomes attenuated and degenerates at week 22 of development because of a reduced blood supply. The term "deciduous" describes a falling off, shedding, or sloughing. The **maternal surface** of the placenta is characterized by 8–10 compartments called **cotyledons** (imparting a **cobblestone appearance**), which are separated by decidual (placental) septa. The maternal surface is **dark red in color and oozes blood** due to torn maternal blood vessels.

2. **The fetal component** of the placenta consists of **tertiary chorionic villi** derived from both the trophoblast and extraembryonic mesoderm, which collectively become known as the **villous chorion.** It develops most prolifically at the site of the decidua basalis. The villous chorion is in contrast to an area of no villous development known as the **smooth chorion** (which is related to the decidua capsularis). The **fetal surface** of the placenta is characterized by the well-vascularized chorionic plate, containing the chorionic (fetal) blood vessels. The fetal surface has a **smooth, shiny, light-blue or blue-pink appearance** (because the amnion covers the fetal surface); 5–8 large chorionic (fetal) blood vessels should be apparent here.

B. Clinical correlations

1. **Velamentous placenta** occurs when the **umbilical (fetal) blood vessels** travel abnormally through the amniochorionic membrane before reaching the placenta proper. If the umbilical (fetal) blood vessels cross the internal os, a serious condition called **vasa previa** exists. If one of the umbilical (fetal) blood vessels ruptures during pregnancy, labor, or delivery in a patient with vasa previa, the fetus will bleed to death.

2. **Placenta previa** occurs when the placenta attaches in the lower part of the uterus, **covering the internal os.** The placenta normally implants in the posterosuperior wall of the uterus. **Uterine (maternal) blood vessels** rupture during the later part of pregnancy as the uterus gradually begins to dilate. As a result, the mother may bleed

A

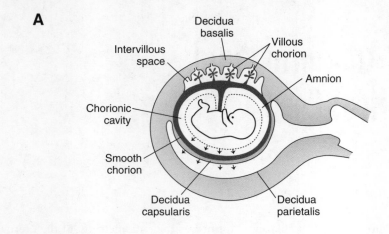

B

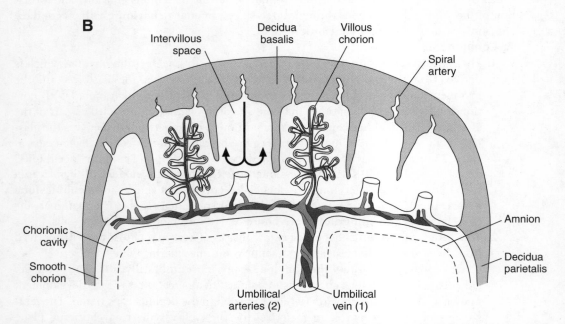

● **Figure 5.1 (A) Relationship of the fetus, uterus, and placenta in the early fetal period.** The small arrows (outer set) indicate that as the fetus grows within the uterine wall, the decidua capsularis expands and fuses with the decidua parietalis, thereby obliterating the uterine cavity. The small arrows (inner set) indicate that as the fetus grows, the amnion expands toward the smooth chorion, thereby obliterating the chorionic cavity. **(B) Diagram of the placenta.** This diagram is oriented in the same direction as (A) for comparison. Note the relationship of the villous chorion (fetal component) to the decidua basalis (maternal component). Maternal blood enters the intervillous space (curved arrow) via the spiral arteries and bathes the villi in maternal blood. The villi contain fetal capillaries and thus maternal/fetal blood exchange occurs.

to death; the fetus will also be placed in jeopardy because of the compromised blood supply. Because the placenta blocks the cervical opening, delivery is usually accomplished by cesarean section. This condition is clinically associated with **repeated episodes of bright red vaginal bleeding.** Placenta previa is the classic cause of **third-trimester bleeding,** whereas an ectopic pregnancy is the classic cause of first-trimester bleeding.

3. **Placenta accreta/increta/percreta** occurs when a placenta implants on the myometrium, deep into the myometrium, or through the wall of the uterus, respectively.

This results in retained placenta and hemorrhage and may lead to uterine rupture (placenta percreta). Risk factors include multiple curettages, previous C-sections, severe endometritis, or closely spaced pregnancies.

4. **Placenta as an allograft.** The fetal component of the placenta inherits both paternal and maternal genes and therefore may be considered as an allograft with respect to the mother. However, the placenta is not rejected in most cases. The two factors responsible for the lack of rejection are as follows:

   a. Syncytiotrophoblast cells lining the villous chorion **lack major histocompatibility (MHC) antigens** and therefore do not evoke an immune response.

   b. Decidual cells within the endometrial stroma secrete **prostaglandin E_2,** which inhibits T-lymphocyte activation.

5. **Preeclampsia and eclampsia.** Severe preeclampsia is the sudden development of **maternal hypertension (>160/110 mm Hg), edema (hands and/or face), and proteinuria (>5 g/24 hr)** usually after week 32 of gestation (third trimester). Eclampsia includes the additional symptom of convulsions. The pathophysiology of preeclampsia involves a **generalized arteriolar constriction** that affects the brain (seizures and stroke), kidneys (oliguria and renal failure), liver (edema), and small blood vessels (thrombocytopenia and disseminated intravascular coagulation). Treatment of severe preeclampsia involves **magnesium sulfate** (for seizure prophylaxis) and **hydralazine** (blood pressure control); once the patient is stabilized, delivery of the fetus should ensue immediately. Risk factors include nulliparity, diabetes, hypertension, renal disease, twin gestation, or hydatidiform mole (produces first-trimester preeclampsia).

II **The Placenta as an Endocrine Organ.** The placenta produces both protein and steroid hormones. **Human chorionic gonadotropin (hCG)** is a glycoprotein hormone that stimulates the production of progesterone by the corpus luteum. **Human placental lactogen (hPL)** is a protein hormone that induces lipolysis, thus elevating the levels of free fatty acid in the mother; it is considered to be the "growth hormone" of the fetus. **Estrone, estradiol (most potent), and estriol** are steroid hormones produced by the placenta, but little is known about their specific functions in either the mother or the fetus. **Progesterone** is a steroid hormone that maintains the endometrium during pregnancy; it is used by the fetal adrenal cortex as a precursor for glucocorticoid and mineralocorticoid synthesis and by the fetal testes as a precursor to testosterone synthesis.

III **The Placental Membrane**

A. **Layers**

   1. In early pregnancy, the placental membrane consists of the **syncytiotrophoblast, cytotrophoblast (Langerhans cells), connective tissue,** and **endothelium of the fetal capillaries. Hofbauer cells** are found in the connective tissue; they are most likely macrophages.

   2. In late pregnancy, the cytotrophoblast degenerates and the connective tissue is displaced by the growth of fetal capillaries, leaving the **syncytiotrophoblast** and the **fetal capillary endothelium.**

B. **Function (Table 5-1).** The **placental membrane** separates maternal blood from fetal blood. A common misperception is that the placental membrane acts as a strict "barrier." However, a wide variety of substances freely cross the placental membrane. Some substances that cross can be either beneficial or harmful. Some substances do not cross the placental membrane. The composition of the placental membrane changes during pregnancy.

C. **Clinical correlation: erythroblastosis fetalis.** The **Rh factor** is clinically important in pregnancy. If the mother is Rh-negative and the fetus is Rh-positive, she will produce

TABLE 5-1	SUBSTANCES THAT CROSS OR DO NOT CROSS THE PLACENTAL MEMBRANE

Beneficial Substances That Cross the Placental Membrane
O_2, CO_2
Glucose, L-form amino acids, free fatty acids, vitamins
H_2O, Na^+, K^+, Ca^{2+}, Cl^-, I^-, PO_4^{2-}
Urea, uric acid, bilirubin1
Fetal and maternal RBCs
Maternal serum proteins, α-fetoprotein, transferrin-Fe^{2+} complex, LDL, prolactin
Steroid hormones (unconjugated)
IgG, IgA

Harmful Substances That Cross the Placental Membrane

Viruses—e.g., rubella, cytomegalovirus, herpes simplex type 2, varicella zoster, coxsackievirus, variola, measles, and poliomyelitis

Category X drugs (absolute contraindication in pregnancy)—e.g., thalidomide, aminopterin, methotrexate, busulfan (Myleran), chlorambucil (Leukeran), cyclophosphamide (Cytoxan), phenytoin (Dilantin), triazolam (Halcion), estazolam (Prosom), warfarin (Coumadin), isotretinoin (Accutane), clomiphene (Clomid), diethylstilbestrol (DES), ethisterone, norethisterone, megestrol (Megace), oral contraceptives (Ovcon, Levlen, Norinyl), nicotine, alcohol, ACE inhibitors (Captopril, Enalapril)

Category D drugs (definite evidence of risk to fetus)—e.g., tetracycline (Achromycin), doxycycline (Vibramycin), streptomycin, Amikacin, tobramycin (Nebcin), phenobarbital (Donnatal), pentobarbital (Nembutal), valproic acid (Depakene), diazepam (Valium), chlordiazepoxide (Librium), alprazolam (Xanax), lorazepam (Ativan), lithium, hydrochlorothiazide (Diuril)
Carbon monoxide
Organic mercury, lead, polychlorinated biphenyls (PCBs), potassium iodide
Cocaine, heroin
Toxoplasma gondii, Treponema pallidum, Listeria monocytogenes
Rubella vaccine
Anti-Rh antibodies

Substances That Do Not Cross the Placental Membrane
Maternally derived cholesterol, triglycerides, and phospholipids
Protein hormones (e.g., insulin)
Drugs (e.g., succinylcholine, curare, heparin, methyldopa, drugs similar to amino acids)
IgD, IgE, IgM
Bacteria in general

Rh antibodies. This situation will not affect the first pregnancy but will affect a second pregnancy with an Rh-positive fetus. Typically the mother becomes sensitized during the first pregnancy. The risk increases in subsequent pregnancies. In the second pregnancy with an Rh-positive fetus, a hemolytic condition of RBCs occurs known as **Rh-hemolytic disease of newborn (erythroblastosis fetalis).** This causes destruction of fetal RBCs, which leads to the release of large amounts of **unconjugated bilirubin** (a breakdown product of hemoglobin). This causes fetal brain damage due to a condition called **kernicterus,** or a pathologic deposition of bilirubin in the basal ganglia. **UV light** is used to treat the newborn with physiological jaundice. **Severe hemolytic disease,** whereby the fetus is severely anemic and demonstrates total body edema (i.e., **hydrops fetalis),** may lead to death. In these cases, an intrauterine transfusion is indicated. **Rh$_0$ immune globulin (Rhogam, MICRhogam)** is a human immunoglobulin (IgG) preparation that contains antibodies against Rh factor and prevents a maternal antibody response to Rh-positive cells that may enter the maternal bloodstream of an Rh-negative mother. This drug is administered to Rh-negative mothers during the third trimester and within 72 hrs after the birth of an Rh-positive baby so as to prevent erythroblastosis fetalis during subsequent pregnancies.

IV **Amniotic Fluid** is maternally derived water that contains electrolytes, carbohydrates, amino acids, lipids, proteins (hormones, enzymes, alpha-fetoprotein), urea, creatinine, lactate, pyruvate, desquamated fetal cells, fetal urine, fetal feces (meconium), and fetal lung liquid (useful for measuring the lecithin/sphingomyelin [L/S] ratio to determine for lung maturity).

A. Production of amniotic fluid. Amniotic fluid is constantly produced during pregnancy by **direct transfer** from maternal circulation in response to osmotic and hydrostatic forces as well as by **excretion of fetal urine by the kidneys** into the amniotic sac. Kidney defects (e.g., bilateral kidney agenesis) result in **oligohydramnios.**

B. Resorption of amniotic fluid. Amniotic fluid is constantly resorbed during pregnancy by the following sequence of events: the fetus swallows amniotic fluid, amniotic fluid is absorbed into fetal blood through the gastrointestinal tract, and excess amniotic fluid is removed via the placenta and passed into maternal blood. Swallowing defects (e.g., esophageal atresia) or absorption defects (e.g., duodenal atresia) result in **polyhydramnios.**

C. The amount of amniotic fluid is gradually increased during pregnancy from **50 mL at week 12** to **1000 mL at term.** The rate of water exchange within the amniotic sac at term is 400–500 mL/hr, with a net flow of 125–200 mL/hr moving from the amniotic fluid into the maternal blood. The near-term fetus excretes about 500 mL of urine daily, which is mostly water, because the placenta exchanges metabolic wastes. The fetus swallows about 400 mL of amniotic fluid daily.

D. Clinical correlations

1. **Oligohydramnios** occurs when there is a low amount of amniotic fluid **(<400 mL in late pregnancy).** Oligohydramnios may be associated with the inability of the fetus to excrete urine into the amniotic sac due to **renal agenesis.** This results in many fetal deformities **(Potter's syndrome)** and **hypoplastic lungs** due to increased pressure on the fetal thorax.

2. **Polyhydramnios** occurs when there is a large amount of amniotic fluid **(>2000 mL in late pregnancy).** Polyhydramnios may be associated with the inability of the fetus to swallow due to **anencephaly, tracheoesophageal fistula,** or **esophageal atresia.** Polyhydramnios is commonly associated with **maternal diabetes.**

3. **α-Fetoprotein (AFP),** or "fetal albumin," is produced by fetal hepatocytes. AFP is routinely assayed in amniotic fluid and maternal serum between **weeks 14–18** of gestation. AFP levels change with gestational age, so that proper interpretation of AFP levels depends on an accurate gestational age. Elevated AFP levels are associated with **neural tube defects** (e.g., **spina bifida or anencephaly), omphalocele** (which allows fetal serum to leak into the amniotic fluid), and **esophageal and duodenal atresia** (which interfere with fetal swallowing). Reduced AFP levels are associated with **Down syndrome.**

4. **Premature rupture of the amniochorionic membrane** is the most common cause of premature labor and oligohydramnios. It is commonly referred to "breaking of the water bag."

5. **Amniotic-band syndrome** occurs when bands of amniotic membrane encircle and constrict parts of the fetus, causing **limb amputations** and **craniofacial anomalies.**

V **Umbilical Cord**

A. Description. There is a patent opening called the **primitive umbilical ring** on the ventral surface of the developing embryo; through it, three structures pass: the **yolk sac (vitelline duct), connecting stalk,** and **allantois.** The allantois is not functional in humans and degenerates to form the **median umbilical ligament** in the adult. As the amnion expands, it pushes the vitelline duct, connecting stalk, and allantois together to form the **primitive umbilical cord.** At week 6, the gut tube connected to the yolk sac will herniate **(physiological umbilical herniation)** into the extraembryonic coelom; the herniation will be reduced by week 11. The gut tube eventually returns to the abdominal cavity, whereas the yolk sac (vitelline duct) and allantois degenerate. The definitive umbilical cord at term is pearly-white, 1–2 cm in diameter, 50–60 cm long, eccentrically positioned, and contains the **right and left umbilical arteries, left umbilical vein,** and **mucous connective tissue (Wharton's jelly).** The right and left umbilical arteries carry deoxygenated blood from the fetus to the placenta. The left umbilical vein carries oxygenated blood from the placenta to the fetus.

B. Clinical correlations

1. **Presence of one umbilical artery** within the umbilical cord is an abnormal finding that suggests cardiovascular abnormalities. Normally, two umbilical arteries are present.

2. **Physical inspection of the umbilicus** in a newborn infant may reveal:

    a. A light-gray shining sac indicating an omphalocele (see Chapter 7).

    b. A fecal (meconium) discharge indicating a vitelline fistula (see Chapter 7).

    c. A urine discharge indicating a urachal fistula (see Chapter 8).

VI **Vasculogenesis (de novo blood vessel formation)** occurs in two general locations, as indicated below.

A. In extraembryonic mesoderm. Vasculogenesis occurs first within extraembryonic visceral mesoderm around the yolk sac on day 17. By day 21, vasculogenesis extends into extraembryonic somatic mesoderm, which is located around the connecting stalk to form the **umbilical vessels,** and in secondary villi to form **tertiary chorionic villi.** Vasculogenesis occurs by a process whereby extraembryonic mesoderm differentiates into **angioblasts,** which form clusters known as **angiogenic cell clusters.** The angioblasts located at the periphery of angiogenic cell clusters give rise to **endothelial cells,** which fuse with each other to form small blood vessels.

B. In intraembryonic mesoderm. Blood vessels form within the embryo by the same mechanism as in extraembryonic mesoderm. Eventually blood vessels formed in the extraembryonic mesoderm become continuous with blood vessels within the embryo, thereby establishing a blood vascular system between the embryo and placenta.

VII **Hematopoiesis (blood cell formation; Figure 5-2).** Hematopoiesis first occurs within the extraembryonic visceral mesoderm around the yolk sac during week 3 of development. During this process, angioblasts within the center of angiogenic cell clusters give rise to primitive blood cells. Beginning at week 5, hematopoiesis is taken over by a sequence of embryonic organs: **liver, spleen, thymus, and bone marrow.**

A. Types of hemoglobin produced during hematopoiesis

1. During the period of yolk sac hematopoiesis, the earliest **embryonic form** of hemoglobin, called **hemoglobin $\delta_2\epsilon_2$,** is synthesized.

2. During the period of liver hematopoiesis, the **fetal form** of hemoglobin (HbF), called **hemoglobin $\alpha_2\gamma_2$,** is synthesized. **Hemoglobin $\alpha_2\gamma_2$** is the predominant form of hemoglobin during pregnancy because it has a higher affinity for oxygen than the **adult form** of hemoglobin (HbA; **hemoglobin $\alpha_2\beta_2$**) and thereby "pulls" oxygen from the maternal blood into fetal blood.

3. During the period of bone marrow hematopoiesis (about week 30), the adult form of hemoglobin is synthesized and gradually replaces **hemoglobin $\alpha_2\gamma_2$.**

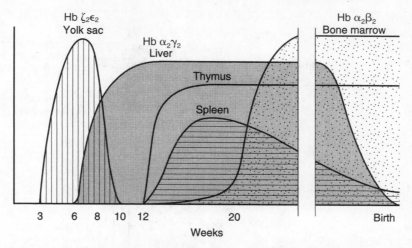

● Figure 5.2 Diagram showing the contribution of various organs to hematopoiesis during embryonic and fetal development.

B. Clinical correlations
   1. Thalassemia syndromes are a heterogeneous group of genetic defects characterized by the lack or decreased synthesis of either the α-globin chain (**α-thalassemia**) or β-globin chain (**β-thalassemia**) of hemoglobin $\alpha_2\beta_2$.
      a. **Hydrops fetalis** is the most severe form of α-thalassemia and causes severe pallor, generalized edema, and massive hepatosplenomegaly. It invariably leads to intrauterine fetal death.
      b. **β-thalassemia major (Cooley anemia)** is the most severe form of β-thalassemia, causing a severe, transfusion-dependent anemia. It is most common in Mediterranean countries and parts of Africa and Southeast Asia.
   2. Hydroxyurea (a cytotoxic drug) has been shown to promote HbF production by the reactivation of γ-chain synthesis. Hydroxyurea has been especially useful in the treatment of **sickle cell disease,** where the presence of HbF counteracts the low oxygen affinity of HbS and inhibits the sickling process.

 Fetal Circulation (**Figure 5-3**). Fetal circulation involves three shunts: the **ductus venosus, ductus arteriosus,** and **foramen ovale.**
   A. Highly oxygenated and nutrient-rich blood returns to the fetus from the placenta via the **left umbilical vein.** (Note: Highly oxygenated blood is carried by the left umbilical vein, not by an artery, as in the adult.) Some blood percolates through the hepatic sinusoids; most of the blood bypasses the sinusoids by passing through the **ductus venosus** and entering the inferior vena cava (IVC). From the IVC, blood enters the right atrium, where most of the blood bypasses the right ventricle through the **foramen ovale** to enter the left atrium. From the left atrium, blood enters the left ventricle and is delivered to fetal tissues via the aorta.
   B. Poorly oxygenated and nutrient-poor fetal blood is sent back to the placenta via the **right and left umbilical arteries.**
   C. Some blood in the right atrium enters the right ventricle; blood in the right ventricle enters the pulmonary trunk, but most of the blood bypasses the lungs through the **ductus arteriosus.** Fetal lungs receive only a minimal amount of blood for growth and development;

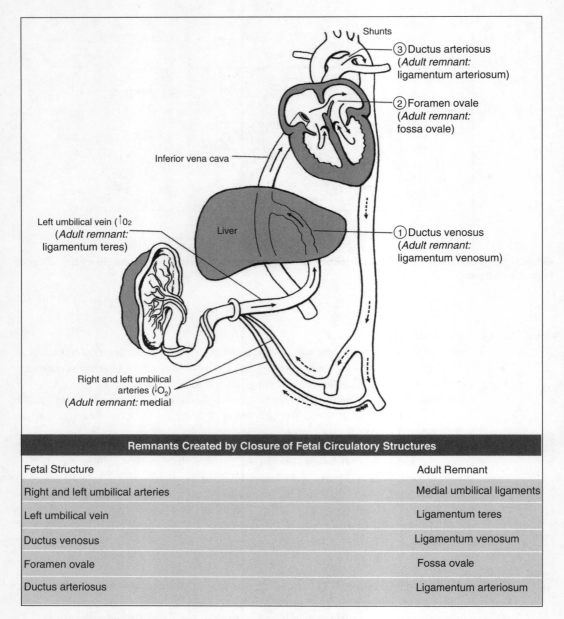

Shunts
③ Ductus arteriosus (*Adult remnant:* ligamentum arteriosum)
② Foramen ovale (*Adult remnant:* fossa ovale)

Inferior vena cava

Left umbilical vein (↑O₂) (*Adult remnant:* ligamentum teres)

Liver

① Ductus venosus (*Adult remnant:* ligamentum venosum)

Right and left umbilical arteries (↓O₂) (*Adult remnant:* medial

Remnants Created by Closure of Fetal Circulatory Structures	
Fetal Structure	Adult Remnant
Right and left umbilical arteries	Medial umbilical ligaments
Left umbilical vein	Ligamentum teres
Ductus venosus	Ligamentum venosum
Foramen ovale	Fossa ovale
Ductus arteriosus	Ligamentum arteriosum

● **Figure 5.3 Fetal circulation.** Note the three shunts and the changes that occur after birth (remnants).

the blood is returned to the left ventricle via the pulmonary veins. Fetal lungs are not capable of performing their adult respiratory function because they are functionally immature and the fetus is under water (surrounded by amnionic fluid). The placenta provides for fetal respiration.

D. Circulatory system changes at birth are facilitated by a **decrease in right atrial pressure** from occlusion of the placental circulation and by an **increase in left atrial pressure** due to increased pulmonary venous return. Changes include closure of the right and left umbilical arteries, left umbilical vein, ductus venosus, ductus arteriosus, and foramen ovale.

Case Study 1

A 37-year-old woman in her third trimester of pregnancy comes in to your clinic complaining of bleeding that lasted for "an hour or two." She says that the bleeding was "very bright red" in color but she felt no noticeable pain. She had done nothing to cause the bleeding and "was concerned for the safety of her baby." What is the most likely diagnosis?

Differentials

• Placenta previa, placenta abruptio, placenta accreta

Relevant Physical Exam Findings

• There was no abdominal or pelvic pain upon palpation.

Relevant Lab Findings

• Transvaginal ultrasound shows an intact, normally implanted placenta. However, the placenta is located in close proximity to the internal os.

Diagnosis

• This is a classic case of placenta previa. The patient is of advanced maternal age and shows bright red bleeding during the third trimester, with the implantation located at or near the internal os. Placental abruption would have shown a separation of the placenta and dark red bleeding accompanied by abdominal pain. Placenta accreta would have shown the placenta implanted much deeper in the myometrium.

Case Study 2

A 34-year-old woman who is in the third trimester of pregnancy complains that her hands and face began "swelling up a few days ago." She also reports that she has felt as though her "heart was racing a mile a minute." What is the most likely diagnosis?

Differentials

• Preeclampsia, renal disease, molar pregnancy

Relevant Physical Exam Findings

• Hypertension
• Hand and facial edema

Relevant Lab Findings

• Proteinuria
• Ultrasound was unremarkable

Diagnosis

• Preeclampsia. The patient's symptoms of hypertension, proteinuria, and edema are all telltale signs of preeclampsia. Also her advancing age has left her susceptible to this condition. Molar pregnancy is normally seen in the first trimester. Renal disease is unlikely because there were no significant findings other than proteinuria.

Chapter 6

Cardiovascular System

I **Formation of the Heart Tube.** Lateral plate mesoderm (at the cephalic area of the embryo) will split into a somatic layer and splanchnic layer, thus forming the **pericardial cavity.** Precardiac mesoderm is preferentially distributed to the splanchnic layer, now becoming known as the **heart-forming regions (HFRs).** As lateral folding of the embryo occurs, the HFRs will fuse in the midline to form a continuous sheet of mesoderm. Hypertrophied foregut endoderm secretes **vascular endothelial growth factor (VEGF),** which induces the sheet of mesoderm to form discontinuous vascular channels that are eventually remodeled into a single **endocardial tube (endocardium).** Mesoderm around the endocardium forms the **myocardium**, which secretes a layer of extracellular matrix proteins called **cardiac jelly.** Mesoderm migrating into the cardiac region from the coelomic wall near the liver forms the **epicardium.**

II **Primitive Heart Tube Dilatations** (**Figure 6-1**). Five dilatations soon become apparent along the length of the tube, namely the **truncus arteriosus, bulbus cordis, primitive ventricle, primitive atrium,** and **sinus venosus.** These five dilatations develop into the adult structures of the heart.

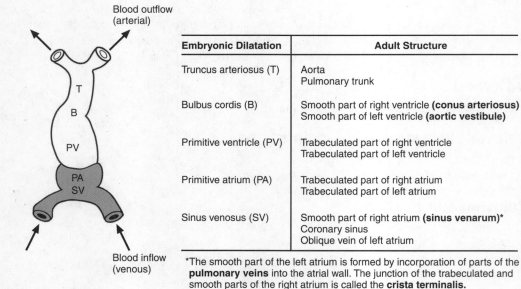

Embryonic Dilatation	Adult Structure
Truncus arteriosus (T)	Aorta Pulmonary trunk
Bulbus cordis (B)	Smooth part of right ventricle **(conus arteriosus)** Smooth part of left ventricle **(aortic vestibule)**
Primitive ventricle (PV)	Trabeculated part of right ventricle Trabeculated part of left ventricle
Primitive atrium (PA)	Trabeculated part of right atrium Trabeculated part of left atrium
Sinus venosus (SV)	Smooth part of right atrium **(sinus venarum)*** Coronary sinus Oblique vein of left atrium

*The smooth part of the left atrium is formed by incorporation of parts of the **pulmonary veins** into the atrial wall. The junction of the trabeculated and smooth parts of the right atrium is called the **crista terminalis.**

● **Figure 6.1 The five dilatations of the heart tube.** T = truncus arteriosus, B = bulbus cordis, PV = primitive ventricle, PA = primitive atrium, SV = sinus venosus. White area: arterial portion. Shaded area: venous portion.

The Aorticopulmonary (AP) Septum (Figure 6-2)

A. Formation. Neural crest cells migrate from the hindbrain region through pharyngeal arches 3, 4, and 6 and invade both the **truncal** and **bulbar ridges.** These ridges grow and twist around one another in a spiral fashion and eventually fuse to form the AP septum. The AP septum divides the truncus arteriosus and bulbus cordis into the aorta and the pulmonary trunk.

B. Clinical correlations

1. **Persistent truncus arteriosus (PTA)** is caused by abnormal neural crest cell migration such that there is only *partial* development of the AP septum. PTA results in a condition in which one large vessel leaves the heart and receives blood from both the right and left ventricles. PTA is usually accompanied by a membranous ventricular septal defect (VSD) and is associated clinically with **marked cyanosis (R→L shunting of blood).**

2. **D-Transposition of the great arteries (complete)** is caused by abnormal neural crest cell migration such that there is *nonspiral* development of the AP septum. D-Transposition results in a condition in which the aorta arises abnormally from the right ventricle and the pulmonary trunk arises abnormally from the left ventricle; hence the systemic and pulmonary circulations are *completely* separated from one another. This condition is incompatible with life unless an accompanying shunt exists, such as a VSD, patent foramen ovale, or patent ductus arteriosus. It is associated clinically with **marked cyanosis (R→L shunting of blood).**

3. **L-Transposition of the great vessels (corrected).** In L-transposition, the aorta and pulmonary trunk are transposed and the ventricles "inverted" such that the anatomical right ventricle lies on the left side and the anatomical left ventricle on the right. These two major deviations offset one another, such that the pattern of blood flow is normal.

4. **Tetralogy of Fallot (TF)** is caused by abnormal neural crest cell migration such that there is *skewed* development of the AP septum. TF results in a condition in which the pulmonary trunk obtains a small diameter while the aorta obtains a large diameter. TF is characterized by four classic malformations: **pulmonary stenosis, right ventricular hypertrophy, overriding aorta, and ventricular septal defect (VSD).** Note the mnemonic **PROVE.** TF is associated clinically with **marked cyanosis (R→L shunting of blood),** the clinical consequences of which depend primarily on the severity of the pulmonary stenosis.

The Atrial Septum (Figure 6-3)

A. Formation. The crescent-shaped **septum primum** forms in the roof of the primitive atrium and grows toward the atrioventricular (AV) cushions in the AV canal. The **foramen primum** forms between the free edge of the septum primum and the AV cushions; it is closed when the septum primum fuses with the AV cushions. The **foramen secundum** forms in the center of the septum primum. The crescent-shaped septum secundum forms to the right of the septum primum. The **foramen ovale** is the opening between the upper and lower limbs of the septum secundum. During embryonic life, blood is shunted from the right atrium to the left atrium via the foramen ovale. Immediately after birth, functional closure of the foramen ovale is facilitated both by a **decrease in right atrial pressure** from occlusion of the placental circulation and by an **increase in left atrial pressure** due to increased pulmonary venous return. Later in life, the septum primum and septum secundum anatomically fuse to complete the formation of the atrial septum.

B. Clinical correlations. Atrial septal defects (ASDs) are noted on auscultation with a loud S_1 and a wide, fixed, split S_2; they are characterized by L→R shunting of blood.

1. **Foramen secundum defect** is caused by excessive resorption of septum primum, septum secundum, or both. This results in a condition in which there is an opening between the right and left atria. Some defects can be tolerated for a long time, with clinical symptoms manifesting as late as age 30. It is the most common clinically significant ASD.

2. **Common atrium (cor triloculare biventriculare)** is caused by the complete failure of septum primum and septum secundum to develop. This results in a condition in which only one atrium is formed.

3. **Probe patency of the foramen ovale** is caused by incomplete anatomic fusion of septum primum and septum secundum. It is present in approximately 25% of the population and is usually of no clinical importance.

4. **Premature closure of foramen ovale** is closure of foramen ovale during prenatal life. It results in hypertrophy of the right side of the heart and underdevelopment of the left side of the heart.

Ⓥ The Atrioventricular (AV) Septum (Figure 6-4)

A. **Formation.** The **dorsal AV cushion** and **ventral AV cushion** approach each other and fuse to form the AV septum. The AV septum partitions the AV canal into the right AV canal and left AV canal.

B. **Clinical correlations**

1. **Persistent common AV canal** is caused by failure of fusion of the dorsal and ventral AV cushions. As a result, the common AV canal is never partitioned into the right and left AV canals, so that a large hole can be found in the center of the heart. Consequently, the tricuspid and bicuspid valves are represented by one valve common to both sides of the heart. Two common hemodynamic abnormalities are found:
   a. L R shunting of blood from the left atrium to the right atrium, causing an enlarged right atrium and right ventricle
   b. Mitral valve regurgitation, causing an enlarged left atrium and left ventricle

2. **Ebstein's anomaly** is caused by failure of the posterior and septal leaflets of the tricuspid valve to attach normally to the annulus fibrosus; they are instead displaced inferiorly into the right ventricle. As a result, the right ventricle is divided into a large upper "atrialized" portion and a small lower functional portion. Because the functional portion of the right ventricle is small, there is less blood available to the pulmonary trunk. This condition is usually associated with an ASD.

3. **Foramen primum defect** is caused by a failure of the AV septum to fuse with the septum primum. It results in a condition in which the foramen primum is never closed and is generally accompanied by an abnormal mitral valve.

4. **Tricuspid atresia (hypoplastic right heart)** is caused when an insufficient amount of AV cushion tissue is available to form the tricuspid valve. The result is complete agenesis of the tricuspid valve, so that there is no communication between the right atrium and right ventricle. It is associated clinically with **marked cyanosis** and is always accompanied by the following:
   a. Patent foramen ovale
   b. IV septum defect
   c. Overdeveloped left ventricle
   d. Underdeveloped right ventricle

The Interventricular (IV) Septum (Figure 6-5)

A. Formation. The muscular IV septum develops in the midline on the floor of the primitive ventricle and grows toward the fused AV cushions. The IV foramen is located between the free edge of the muscular IV septum and the fused AV cushions. This foramen is closed by the membranous IV septum, which forms by the proliferation and fusion of tissue from three sources: the right bulbar ridge, left bulbar ridge, and AV cushions.

B. Clinical correlations. IV septal defects (VSDs)

1. **Membranous VSD** is caused by faulty fusion of the **right bulbar ridge, left bulbar ridge,** and **AV cushions.** As a result, an opening between the right and left ventricles allows free flow of blood. A large VSD is initially associated with L→R shunting of blood, increased pulmonary blood flow, and pulmonary hypertension. Patients with L→R shunting of blood complain of **excessive fatigue on exertion.**

2. **Eisenmenger syndrome (uncorrected VSD, ASD, or PDA).** Initially, a VSD, ASD, or PDA is associated with L→R shunting of blood, increased pulmonary blood flow, and pulmonary hypertension. Later, the pulmonary hypertension causes marked proliferation of the tunica intima and tunica media of pulmonary muscular arteries and arterioles, resulting in a narrowing of their lumens. Ultimately, pulmonary resistance may become higher than systemic resistance and cause **R→L shunting** of blood and **cyanosis.**

3. **Muscular VSD** is caused by single or multiple perforations in the muscular IV septum.

4. **Common ventricle (cor triloculare biatriatum)** is caused by failure of the membranous and muscular IV septa to form.

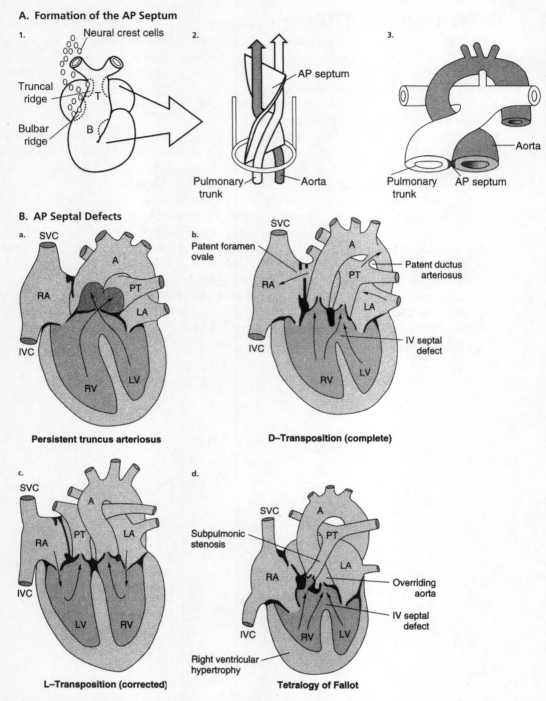

A. Formation of the AP Septum

1.
Neural crest cells

Truncal ridge

Bulbar ridge

T

B

2.
AP septum

Pulmonary trunk   Aorta

3.
Aorta

Pulmonary trunk   AP septum

B. AP Septal Defects

a.
SVC

A

RA

PT

LA

IVC

RV   LV

Persistent truncus arteriosus

b.
SVC

Patent foramen ovale

RA

A

PT

Patent ductus arteriosus

LA

IVC

IV septal defect

RV   LV

D–Transposition (complete)

c.
SVC

A

RA   PT   LA

IVC

LV   RV

L–Transposition (corrected)

d.
SVC

A

Subpulmonic stenosis

RA

PT

LA

Overriding aorta

IV septal defect

IVC

RV   LV

Right ventricular hypertrophy

Tetralogy of Fallot

● **Figure 6.2 (A) Formation of the AP septum, 1 to 3. (B) AP septal defects.** (a) Persistent truncus arteriosus. (b) D-Transposition of the great arteries (complete). (c) L-Transposition of the great arteries. (d) Tetralogy of Fallot.

A. Formation of the Atrial Septum

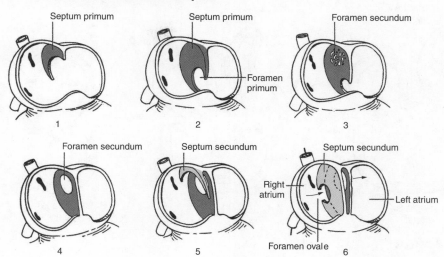

B. Atrial Septal Defects (ASDs)

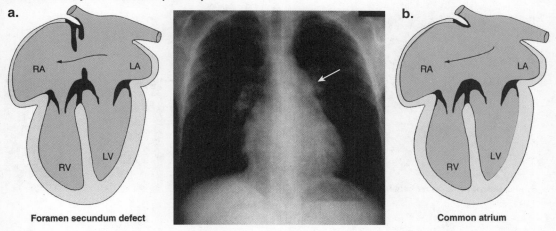

● **Figure 6.3 (A) Formation of the atrial septum, 1 to 6.** The arrows in part 6 indicate the direction of blood flow across the fully developed septum, from the right atrium to the left atrium. **(B) Atrial septal defects (ASDs).** (a) Foramen secundum defect. The AP radiograph of a foramen secundum defect shows cardiomegaly due to en-largement of the right atrium and right ventricle (the left atrium and ventricle is generally of normal size), enlargement of the pulmonary artery (arrow), and increased pulmonary vascularity. The enlarged pulmonary arteries prevent the aorta from forming the normal left border of the heart (i.e., the aortic knob is small). (b) Common atrium. Arrows indicate the direction of blood flow. LA = left atrium; LV = left ventricle; RA = right atrium; RV = right ventricle.

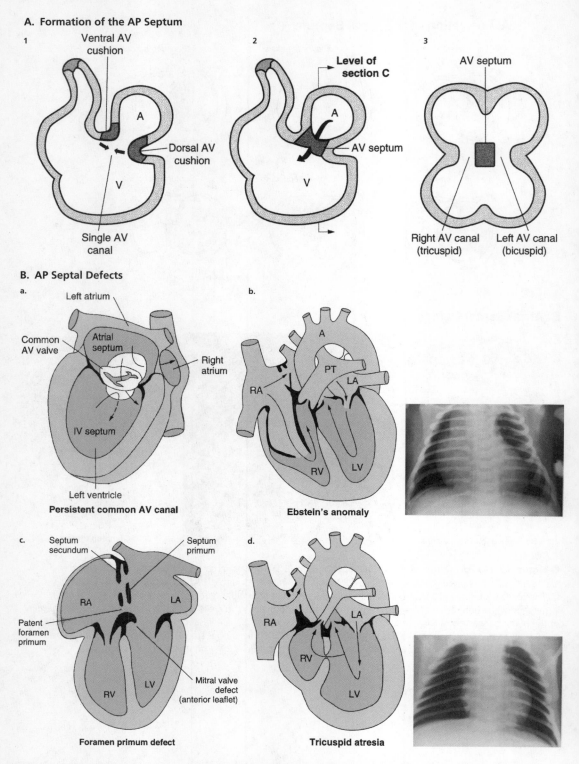

A. Formation of the AP Septum

1
Ventral AV cushion
A
Dorsal AV cushion
Single AV canal

2
Level of section C
A
AV septum
V

3
AV septum
Right AV canal (tricuspid)
Left AV canal (bicuspid)

B. AP Septal Defects

a.
Left atrium
Common AV valve
Atrial septum
Right atrium
IV septum
Left ventricle
Persistent common AV canal

b.
A
PT
LA
RA
RV
LV
Ebstein's anomaly

c.
Septum secundum
Septum primum
RA
LA
Patent foramen primum
Mitral valve defect (anterior leaflet)
RV
LV
Foramen primum defect

d.
RA
LA
RV
LV
Tricuspid atresia

● **Figure 6.4 (A) Formation of the AV septum (1 to 3), which partitions the atrioventricular canal. (B) AV septal defects.** (a) Persistent common AV canal. (b) Ebstein's anomaly. AP radiograph shows massive cardiomegaly due to enlargement of the right atrium. The left cardiac contour is also abnormal due to displacement of the right ventricular outflow tract. (c) Foramen primum defect. (d) Tricuspid atresia. The AP radiograph shows a normal-sized heart with a convex left cardiac contour. Arrows indicate the direction of blood flow. A = atrium (A), V = ventricle, AV = atrioventricular. A = aorta (B), LA = left atrium, LV = left ventricle, RA = right atrium, RV = right ventricle, PT = pulmonary trunk.

A. Formation of IV Septum

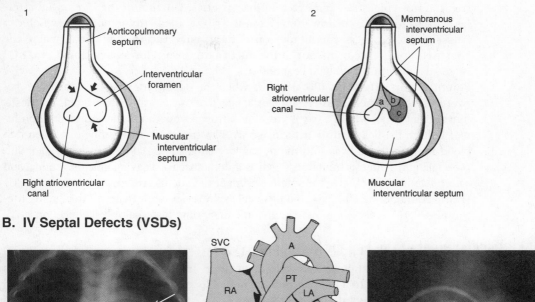

● **Figure 6.5 (A) Formation of the IV septum (1 and 2), which partitions the primitive ventricle.** The shaded portion (a, b, c) in part 2 indicates the three sources of the membranous interventricular septum: a = right bulbar ridge, b = left bulbar ridge, c = AV cushions. **(B) IV septal defects (VSDs).** A membranous VSD is shown. The AP radiograph demonstrates cardiomegaly and a marked enlargement of the main pulmonary artery (arrow). Left ventriculography in the LAO position demonstrates flow of contrast material from the left ventricle (LV) through a membranous VSD into the right ventricle (RV). Arrows indicate the direction of blood flow. A = aorta, LA = left atrium, LV = left ventricle, RA = right atrium, RV = right ventricle, PT = pulmonary trunk, IVC inferior vena cava, SVC = superior vena cava.

VII Development of the Arterial System (Table 6-1)

A. Formation. In the head and neck region, the arterial pattern develops mainly from six pairs of arteries (called **aortic arches**) that course through the pharyngeal arches. The aortic arch arteries undergo a complex remodeling process that results in the adult arterial pattern. In the rest of the body, the arterial patterns develop mainly from the **right and left dorsal aortae.** The right and left dorsal aortae fuse to form the **dorsal aorta,** which then sprouts **posterolateral arteries, lateral arteries,** and **ventral arteries (vitelline and umbilical).**

B. Clinical correlations

1. Postductal coarctation of the aorta occurs when the aorta is abnormally constricted. A postductal coarctation is found distal to the origin of the left subclavian artery and inferior to the ductus arteriosus. It is clinically associated with increased blood pressure in the upper extremities, lack of pulse in femoral artery, and a high risk of both cerebral hemorrhage and bacterial endocarditis. Collateral circulation around the constriction involves the internal thoracic, intercostal, superior epigastric, inferior epigastric, and external iliac arteries. Dilation of the intercostal arteries causes erosion of the lower border of the ribs (called "rib notching"), which can be seen on x-ray. Less commonly, a **preductal coarctation** may occur, where the constriction is located superior to the ductus arteriosus. Turner syndrome (45, XO) is associated with a preductal coarctation.

2. **Patent ductus arteriosus (PDA)** occurs when the ductus arteriosus, a connection between the left pulmonary artery and aorta, fails to close. Normally the ductus arteriosus functionally closes within a few hours after birth via smooth muscle contraction to ultimately form the **ligamentum arteriosum.** A PDA causes L→R shunting of oxygen-rich blood from the aorta back into the pulmonary circulation. A PDA can be treated with prostaglandin synthesis inhibitors (such as indomethacin), acetylcholine, histamine, and catecholamines, all of which promote closure of the ductus arteriosus. Prostaglandin E1 (PGE_1), intrauterine asphyxia, and neonatal asphyxia sustain patency of the ductus arteriosus. A PDA is very common in premature infants and maternal rubella infection.

 Development of the Venous System (**Table 6-1**).   The venous system develops from the **vitelline, umbilical,** and **cardinal veins** that empty into the sinus venosus. These veins undergo remodeling due to a redirection of venous blood from the left side of the body to the right in order to empty into the right atrium.

TABLE 6-1	DEVELOPMENT OF THE ARTERIAL AND VENOUS SYSTEMS
Embryonic Structure	**Adult Structure**
Aortic arches	
1	Maxillary artery (portion of)
2	Stapedial artery (portion of)
3	R & L common carotid arteries (portion of)
	R & L internal carotid arteries
4	Right subclavian artery (portion of)
	Arch of the aorta (portion of)
5	Regresses in the human
6*	R & L pulmonary arteries (portion of)
	Ductus arteriosus
Dorsal aorta	
Posterolateral branches	Arteries to upper and lower extremities
	Intercostal, lumbar, and lateral sacral arteries
Lateral branches	Renal, suprarenal, and gonadal arteries
Ventral branches	
Vitelline arteries	Celiac, superior mesenteric, and inferior mesenteric arteries
Umbilical arteries	Internal iliac arteries (portion of), superior vesical arteries
	Medial umbilical ligaments
Vitelline veins	
Right and left	Portion of the IVC,† hepatic veins and sinusoids, ductus venosus, portal vein,
	inferior mesenteric vein, superior mesenteric vein, splenic vein
Umbilical veins	
Right	Hepatic sinusoids (degenerates early in fetal life)
Left	Hepatic sinusoids, ligamentum teres
Cardinal veins	
Anterior	SVC, internal jugular veins
Posterior	Portion of IVC, common iliac veins
Subcardinal	Portion of IVC, renal veins, gonadal veins
Supracardinal	Portion of IVC, intercostal veins, hemiazygos vein, azygos vein

*Early in development, the recurrent laryngeal nerves hook around aortic arch 6. On the right side, the distal part of aortic arch 6 regresses, and the right recurrent laryngeal nerve moves up to hook around the right subclavian artery. On the left side, aortic arch 6 persists as the ductus arteriosus (or ligamentum arteriosus in the adult); the left recurrent laryngeal nerve remains hooked around the ductus arteriosus.

†IVC = inferior vena cava. Note that the IVC is derived embryologically from four different sources. SVC = superior vena cava.

Case Study

A distraught father comes in with his 10-year-old son saying that his son began "turning blue" when they were out playing catch. His son remarked that he "just felt really tired" when he was running after the ball. The father is concerned that his son would not be able to play in the big game this weekend. What is the most likely diagnosis?

Differentials

- Congenital septal defect (ASD, VSD, PDA), Eisenmenger's complex, coarctation of the aorta, asthma

Relevant Physical Exam Findings

- Loud holosystolic ejection murmur on auscultation
- Cyanosis
- Clubbing of fingernails

Relevant Lab Findings

- ECG shows right ventricular hypertrophy.

Diagnosis

- VSD. Upon auscultation, the child is found to have a holosystolic murmur, which can result over time in an Eisenmenger complex—that is, a shift from a left-to-right shunt to a right-to-left shunt. In this instance the symptom of cyanosis became apparent in childhood rather than infancy. An ASD would have a fixed split S_2 systolic ejection murmur. A PDA, which is normally detected in infants, would have a continuous machine-like murmur. Coarctation of the aorta would show a holosystolic murmur; however, there was no finding of a lack of a femoral pulse or of rib notching.

Chapter 7

Digestive System

❶ **Primitive Gut Tube** (**Figure 7-1**). The **primitive gut tube** is formed from the incorpo-ration of the dorsal part of the yolk sac into the embryo due to the craniocaudal folding and lateral folding of the embryo. The primitive gut tube extends from the oropharyngeal membrane to the cloacal membrane and is divided into the **foregut, midgut,** and **hindgut.** Histologically, the general plan of the adult gastrointestinal tract consists of a **mucosa** (epithelial lining and glands, lamina propria, and muscularis mucosae), **submucosa, muscularis externa,** and **adventitia** or **serosa.** Embryologically, the epithelial lining and glands of the mucosa are derived from endoderm, whereas the other components are derived from visceral mesoderm. Early in development, the epithelial lining of the gut tube proliferates rapidly and obliterates the lumen. Later, **recanalization** occurs.

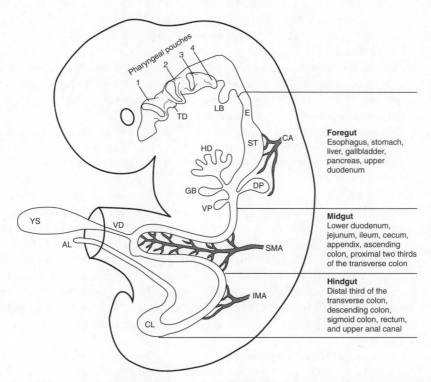

● **Figure 7.1 Development of the gastrointestinal tract, showing the foregut, midgut, and hindgut along with the adult derivatives.** The entire length of the endodermal gut tube is shown from the mouth to the anus. The fate of the lung bud (LB) is covered in Chapter 10. The fate of the pharyngeal pouches (1 to 4) and thyroid diverticulum (TD) is covered in Chapter 11. E = esophagus, ST = stomach, HD = hepatic diverticulum, GB = gallbladder, VP = ventral pancreatic bud, DP = dorsal pancreatic bud, CA = celiac artery, YS = yolk sac, VD = vitelline duct, AL = allantois, SMA = superior mesenteric artery, CL = cloaca, IMA = inferior mesenteric artery.

Foregut Derivatives are supplied by the **celiac artery.**

A. Esophagus (Figure 7-2)

1. **Formation.** The foregut is divided into the esophagus dorsally and the trachea ventrally by the **tracheoesophageal folds,** which fuse to form the **tracheoesophageal septum.** The esophagus is initially short but lengthens with descent of the heart and lungs. During development, the endodermal lining of the esophagus proliferates rapidly and obliterates the lumen; later, recanalization occurs.

2. **Clinical correlations**

   a. **Esophageal atresia** occurs when the tracheoesophageal septum deviates too far dorsally, causing the esophagus to end as a closed tube. About 33% of patients with esophageal atresia also have other congenital defects associated with the VATER or VACTERL syndromes. Esophageal atresia is associated clinically with polyhydramnios (the fetus is unable to swallow amniotic fluid) and a tracheoesophageal fistula.

   b. **Esophageal stenosis** occurs when the lumen of the esophagus is narrowed; it usually involves the midesophagus. The stenosis may be caused by hypertrophy of the submucosal/muscularis externa, remnants of the tracheal cartilaginous ring within the wall of the esophagus, or a membranous diaphragm obstructing the lumen, probably due to incomplete recanalization.

   c. **Esophageal duplication** occurs most commonly due to a congenital esophageal cyst, which is usually found (in 60% of the cases) in the lower esophagus. Duplication cysts may lie on the posterior aspect of the esophagus, where they protrude into the posterior mediastinum or within the wall of the esophagus (i.e., they are intramural).

   d. **Vascular compression of the esophagus** occurs when there is an abnormal origin of the **right subclavian artery** due to developmental anomalies of the aortic arches. The anomalous right subclavian artery passes from the aortic arch behind the esophagus and may cause dysphagia ("dysphagia lusoria").

   e. **Achalasia** occurs due to the loss of ganglion cells in the myenteric (Auerbach) plexus and is characterized by failure to relax the lower esophageal sphincter, which causes progressive dysphagia and difficulty in swallowing.

B. Stomach (Figure 7-3)

1. **Formation.** In week 4, a fusiform dilatation forms in the foregut, which gives rise to the **primitive stomach.** The dorsal part of the primitive stomach grows faster than the ventral part, thereby resulting in the greater and lesser curvatures, respectively. The primitive stomach rotates 90° clockwise around its longitudinal axis. The 90° rotation affects all foregut structures and is responsible for the adult anatomic relationship of foregut viscera. As a result of this clockwise rotation, the dorsal mesentery is carried to the left and eventually forms the **greater omentum;** the **left vagus nerve (CN X)** innervates the ventral surface of the stomach; and the **right vagus nerve (CN X)** innervates the dorsal surface of the stomach.

2. **Clinical correlation. Hypertrophic pyloric stenosis** occurs when the muscularis externa in the pyloric region hypertrophies, causing a narrow pyloric lumen that obstructs the passage of food. It is associated clinically with projectile, nonbilious vomiting after feeding and a small palpable mass at the right costal margin; increased incidence has been found in infants treated with the antibiotic erythromycin. Treatment involves surgical incision of the hypertrophic muscle.

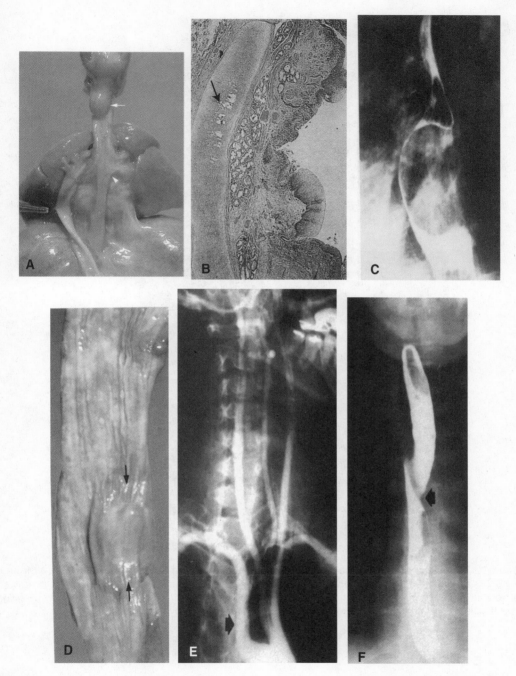

● **Figure 7.2 (A) Esophageal atresia.** A posterior view shows that the esophagus terminates blindly in a blunted esophageal pouch (arrow). There is a distal esophageal connection with the trachea at the carina (arrowhead). **(B) Esophageal stenosis.** This micrograph shows the stratified squamous epithelial lining of the esophagus and submucosal glands. Note that a portion of the muscular wall contains remnants of cartilage (arrow), which contribute to a stenosis. **(C,D) Esophageal duplication cyst.** A barium esophagram demonstrates a large intramural duplication cyst in the proximal esophagus. The cyst shows acute angles with the esophageal lumen, indicating its intramural location. A gross anatomy photograph of the esophagus shows a large intramural duplication cyst (arrows). **(E,F) Vascular compression of the esophagus.** An angiogram reveals an anomalous right subclavian artery (arrow) arising from the aortic arch. A barium esophagram in the same patient reveals an oblique compression of the esophagus (arrow) due to the anomalous right subclavian artery.

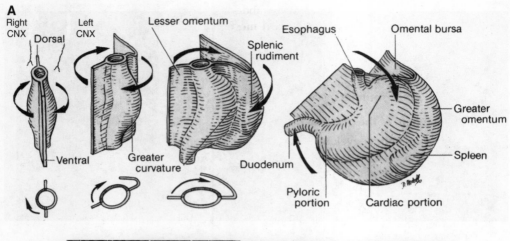

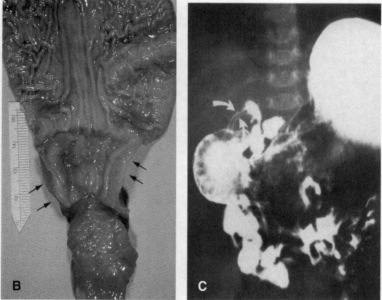

● **Figure 7.3 (A) Diagram depicting the development and 90° rotation of the stomach from week 4 through week 6. (B,C) Hypertrophic pyloric stenosis.** A gross photograph of the stomach opened along the greater curvature. Note the prominence of the pyloric ring, indicated by the arrows. A barium contrast radiograph shows the long, narrow double channel of the pylorus (arrows) in a patient with hypertrophic pyloric stenosis.

C. Liver

1. **Formation.** The endodermal lining of the foregut forms an outgrowth (called the **hepatic diverticulum**) into the surrounding mesoderm of the **septum transversum**. The mesoderm of the septum transversum is involved in the formation of the **diaphragm,** which explains the intimate gross anatomic relationship between the liver and diaphragm. Cords of hepatoblasts (called **hepatic cords**) from the hepatic diverticulum grow into the mesoderm of the septum transversum, where critical hepatoblast/mesoderm interactions occur. The hepatic cords arrange themselves around the **vitelline veins and umbilical veins,** which course through the septum transversum and form the **hepatic sinusoids.** Due to the tremendous growth of the

liver, the liver bulges into the abdominal cavity, thereby stretching the septum transversum to form the **ventral mesentery,** consisting of the **falciform ligament** and the **lesser omentum.** The falciform ligament contains the **left umbilical vein,** which regresses after birth to form the **ligamentum teres.** The lesser omentum can be divided into the **hepatogastric ligament** and the **hepatoduodenal ligament.** The hepatoduodenal ligament contains the **bile duct, portal vein, and hepatic artery (i.e., the portal triad).**

2. **Clinical correlation.** Congenital malformations of the liver are rare.

D. Gallbladder and bile ducts (Figure 7-4)

1. **Formation.** The connection between the hepatic diverticulum and the foregut narrows to form the bile duct. An outgrowth from the bile duct gives rise to the **gallbladder rudiment** and **cystic duct.** The cystic duct divides the bile duct into the common hepatic duct and common bile duct. During development, the endodermal lining of the gallbladder and extrahepatic bile ducts proliferates rapidly and obliterates the lumen; later, recanalization occurs.

2. **Clinical Correlations**

   a. **Intrahepatic gallbladder** occurs when the gallbladder rudiment advances beyond the hepatic diverticulum and becomes buried within the substance of the liver.

   b. **Floating gallbladder** occurs when the gallbladder rudiment lags behind the hepatic diverticulum and thereby becomes suspended from the liver by a mesentery. A floating gallbladder is at risk for **torsion.**

   c. **Developmental anomalies of the cystic duct's** anatomy are fairly common.

   d. **Developmental anomalies of the gallbladder's** anatomy are fairly common, whereby two bilobed diverticula and septated gallbladders are found.

   e. **Biliary atresia** is defined as the obliteration of extrahepatic and/or intrahepatic ducts. Due to acute and chronic inflammation, the ducts are replaced by fibrotic tissue. This condition is associated clinically with progressive neonatal jaundice beginning soon after birth, white or clay-colored stool, and dark urine. The average survival time is 12–19 months, with a 100% mortality rate.

E. Pancreas (Figure 7-5)

1. **Formation.** The **dorsal pancreatic bud** is a direct outgrowth of foregut endoderm, whose formation is induced by the notochord. The **ventral pancreatic bud** is a direct outgrowth of foregut endoderm whose formation is induced by hepatic mesoderm. Within both pancreatic buds, endodermal tubules surrounded by mesoderm branch repeatedly to form acinar cells and ducts (i.e., exocrine pancreas). Isolated clumps of endodermal cells bud from the tubules and accumulate within the mesoderm to form **islet cells** (i.e., endocrine pancreas) in the following sequence (first→last): **alpha cells** (glucagon)→ **beta cells** (insulin)→ **delta cells** (somatostatin) and **PP cells** (pancreatic polypeptide). Because of the 90-degree clockwise rotation of the duodenum, the ventral bud rotates dorsally and fuses with the dorsal bud to form the definitive adult pancreas. The ventral bud forms the **uncinate process** and a **portion of the head of the pancreas.** The dorsal bud forms the **remaining portion of the head, body,** and **tail of the pancreas.** The main pancreatic duct is formed by the anastomosis of the **distal two-thirds of the dorsal pancreatic duct** (the proximal third regresses) and the **entire ventral pancreatic duct** (48% incidence). The main pancreatic duct and common bile duct form a single opening (**hepatopancreatic ampulla of Vater**) into the duodenum at the tip of a major papilla (**hepatopancreatic papilla**). The **ventral pancreatic bud** forms the uncinate process and part of the head of the pancreas. The **dorsal pancreatic bud** forms the remaining part of the head, body, and tail of the pancreas. Acinar cells, ductal epithelium, and islet cells are derived from endoderm.

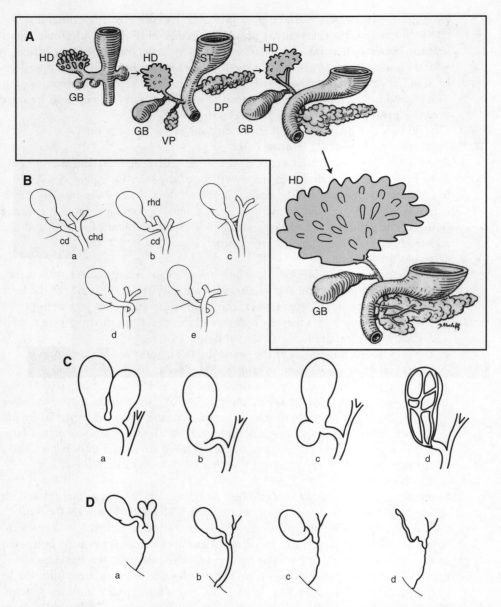

● **Figure 7.4 (A) Sequence of events in the development of the hepatic diverticulum (HD) and gallbladder rudiment (GB) from week 4 through week 7. (B) Developmental anomalies of the cystic duct.** (a) The cystic duct (cd) joins the common hepatic duct (chd) directly (most common anatomical arrangement). (b) The cystic duct joins the right hepatic duct (rhd). (c) Low junction of the cystic duct with the common hepatic duct. (d) Anterior spiral of the cystic duct. (e) Posterior spiral of the cystic duct. **(C) Developmental anomalies of the gallbladder.** (a) Two gallbladders. (b) Bilobed gallbladder. (c) Diverticulum of the gallbladder. (d) Septated gallbladder, which is most likely due to incomplete recanalization of the lumen. **(D) Different forms of extrahepatic biliary atresia.** (a to c) Partial. (d) Complete.

2. Clinical correlations

a. **The accessory pancreatic duct** develops when the proximal third of the dorsal pancreatic duct persists and opens into the duodenum through a minor papilla at a site proximal to the ampulla of Vater (33% incidence).

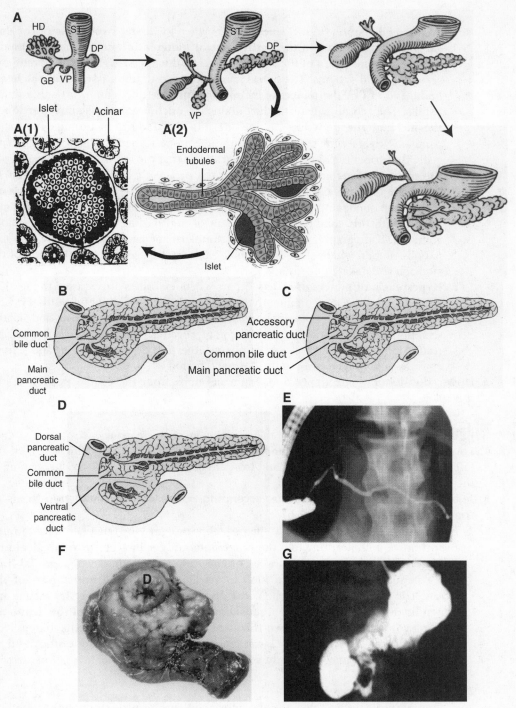

● **Figure 7.5 (A) Sequence of events in the development of the pancreatic buds from weeks 4 through 7.** Note that, within the pancreatic buds, endodermal tubules branch repeatedly to form the exocrine (acinar) pancreas. Islets bud from the endodermal tubules to form the endocrine (islet) pancreas. HD = hepatic diverticulum, GB = gallbladder rudiment, VP = ventral pancreatic bud, DP = dorsal pancreatic bud, ST = stomach. **(B) Normal pattern of the main pancreatic duct (48% incidence in the population). (C) Accessory pancreatic duct (33% incidence in the population).** Note that the proximal third of the dorsal pancreatic duct persists. **(D,E) Pancreas divisum.** Note that the distal two thirds of the dorsal and ventral pancreatic ducts fail to anastomose, thereby forming two separate duct systems. An endoscopic retrograde pancreatogram performed through the accessory minor papillae shows the dorsal pancreatic duct in pancreatic divisum. **(F,G) Annular pancreas.** Photograph of a pathological specimen showing a ring of pancreatic tissue surrounding the entire duodenum (D). Barium contrast radiograph showing partial duodenal obstruction consistent with an annular pancreas.

b. **Pancreas divisum** (4% incidence) occurs when the **distal two-thirds of the dorsal pancreatic duct** and the **entire ventral pancreatic duct** fail to anastomose and the proximal third of the dorsal pancreatic duct persists, thereby forming two separate ductal systems. The dorsal pancreatic duct drains a **portion of the head, body,** and **tail of the pancreas** by opening into the duodenum through a minor papilla. The ventral pancreatic duct drains the **uncinate process** and a **portion of the head of the pancreas** by opening into the duodenum through the major papilla. Patients with pancreas divisum are prone to develop pancreatitis, especially if the opening of the dorsal pancreatic duct at the minor papilla is small.

c. **Annular pancreas** occurs when the ventral pancreatic bud fuses with the dorsal bud both dorsally and ventrally, thereby forming a **ring of pancreatic tissue** around the duodenum and causing severe **duodenal obstruction.** Newborns and infants with this condition are intolerant of oral feeding and often have bilious vomiting. Radiographic evidence of an annular pancreas is indicated by a duodenal obstruction where a "double bubble" sign is often seen, due to dilation of the stomach and distal duodenum.

d. **Hyperplasia of pancreatic islets** occurs when fetal islets are exposed to high levels of blood glucose, as frequently happens in **infants of diabetic mothers.** Glucose freely crosses the placenta and stimulates fetal islet hyperplasia and insulin secretion, which causes increased fat and glycogen deposition in fetal tissues. This results in increased birth weight of infants at term (i.e., **macrosomia**) and serious episodes of **hypoglycemia** in the postnatal period.

F. **Upper duodenum.** The upper duodenum develops from the caudal portion of the foregut.

III   Midgut Derivatives are supplied by the **superior mesenteric artery.**

A. **Lower duodenum.** The **lower duodenum** develops from the cranialmost part of the midgut. The junction of the upper and lower duodenum is just distal to the opening of the common bile duct.

B. **Jejunum, ileum, cecum, appendix, ascending colon, and proximal two-thirds of the transverse colon (Figure 7-6)**

1. **Formation.** The midgut forms a U-shaped loop (**midgut loop**) that herniates through the primitive umbilical ring into the extraembryonic coelom (i.e., **physiological umbilical herniation**) beginning at week 6. The midgut loop consists of a **cranial limb** and a **caudal limb.** The cranial limb forms the **jejunum** and **upper part of the ileum.** The caudal limb forms the **cecal diverticulum,** from which the **cecum** and **appendix** develop; the rest of the caudal limb forms the **lower part of the ileum, ascending colon,** and **proximal two-thirds of the transverse colon.** The midgut loop rotates a total of 270° counterclockwise around the superior mesenteric artery as it returns to the abdominal cavity, thus reducing the physiological herniation, around week 11.

2. **Clinical correlations**

a. **Omphalocele** occurs when the abdominal contents herniate through the umbilical ring and persist outside the body, covered variably by a translucent peritoneal membrane sac (a light-gray shiny sac) protruding from the base of the umbilical cord. Large omphaloceles may contain stomach, liver, and intestines. Small omphaloceles contain only intestines. Omphaloceles are usually associated with other congenital anomalies (e.g., trisomy 13, trisomy 18, or Beckwith-Wiedemann syndrome).

b. **Gastroschisis** occurs when there is a defect in the ventral abdominal wall, usually to the right of the umbilical ring, through which there is a massive evisceration of

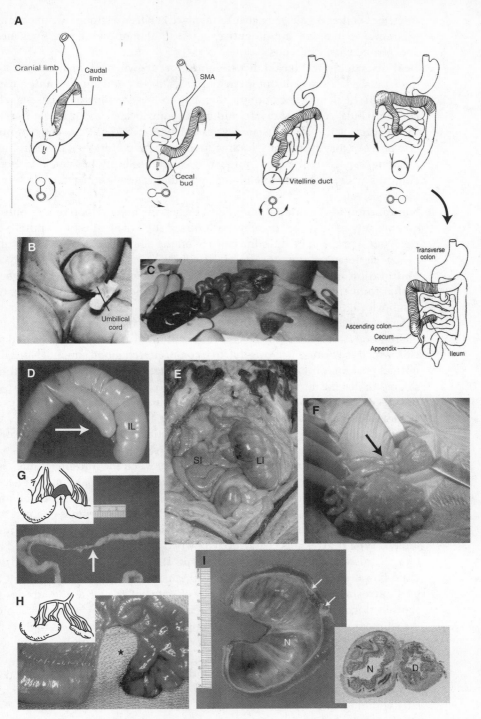

● **Figure 7.6 (A) Diagram depicting the 270° counterclockwise rotation of the midgut loop.** Striped area indicates the caudal limb. Note that after the 270° rotation, the cecum and appendix are located in the upper abdominal cavity. Later in development, there is growth in the direction indicated by the bold arrow, so that the cecum and appendix end up in the lower right quadrant. **(B) Omphalocele. (C) Gastroschisis. (D) Meckel diverticulum (arrow). (E) Nonrotation of midgut loop.** Note small intestines (SI) on the right side and large intestines (LI) on left side. **(F) Volvulus.** Note the twisting (arrow) of the small intestines around the axis of the mesentery. **(G) Type II atresia.** Note the fibrous cord (arrow). **(H) Type IIIa atresia.** Note the gap in the mesentery (∗). **(I) Duplication.** Note the larger diameter of the normal bowel segment (N) and the smaller diameter of the duplicated segment (D). Atretic areas (arrows) are indicated in the duplicated segment.

intestines (other organs may also be involved). The intestines are not covered by a peritoneal membrane, are directly exposed to amniotic fluid, are thickened, and are covered with adhesions.

c. **Ileal diverticulum (Meckel diverticulum)** occurs when a remnant of the vitelline duct persists, thereby forming an outpouching located on the **antemesenteric border** of the ileum. The outpouching may connect to the umbilicus via a fibrous cord or fistula. A Meckel diverticulum is usually located about 30 cm proximal to the ileocecal valve in infants and varies in length from 2–15 cm. **Heterotopic gastric mucosa** may be present, leading to ulceration, perforation, or gastrointestinal bleeding, especially if a large number of parietal cells are present. It is associated clinically with symptoms resembling appendicitis and bright-red or dark-red (i.e., bloody) stools.

d. **Nonrotation of the midgut loop** occurs when the midgut loop rotates only 90 degrees counterclockwise, thereby positioning the small intestine entirely on the right side and the large intestine entirely on the left, with the cecum located either in the left upper quadrant or the left iliac fossa.

e. **Malrotation of the midgut loop** occurs when the midgut loop undergoes only partial counterclockwise rotation. This results in the cecum and appendix lying in a subpyloric or subhepatic location and the small intestine suspended by only a vascular pedicle (i.e., not a broad mesentery). A major clinical complication of malrotation is **volvulus** (twisting of the small intestines around the vascular pedicle), which may cause necrosis due to a compromised blood supply. (Note: The abnormal position of the appendix due to malrotation of the midgut should be considered in diagnosing appendicitis.)

f. **Reversed rotation of the midgut loop** occurs when the midgut loop rotates clockwise instead of counterclockwise, causing the large intestine to enter the abdominal cavity first. This causes the large intestine to be anatomically located posterior to the duodenum and superior mesenteric artery.

g. **Intestinal atresia and stenosis.** Atresia occurs when the intestinal lumen is completely occluded; whereas stenosis occurs when the intestinal lumen is narrowed. The causes of these conditions seem to be both failed recanalization and/or an ischemic intrauterine event ("vascular accident"). **Type I atresia** is characterized by a membranous septum or diaphragm of mucosa and submucosa that obstructs the lumen. **Type II atresia** is characterized by two blind bowel ends connected by a fibrous cord with an intact mesentery. **Type IIIa atresia** is characterized by two blind bowel ends separated by a gap in the mesentery. **Type IIIb atresia ("apple peel" atresia)** is characterized by a bowel segment (distal to the atresia) that is shortened, coiled around a mesentery remnant, and lacking a blood supply from the superior mesenteric artery (blood supply to this bowel segment is via collateral circulation). **Type IV atresia** is characterized by multiple atresias throughout the bowel, having the appearance of a "string of sausages." Proximal atresias are associated clinically with polyhydramnios and bilious vomiting soon after birth. Distal atresias are associated clinically with normal amniotic fluid, abdominal distention, later vomiting, and failure to pass meconium.

h. **Duplication of the intestines** occurs when a segment of the intestines is duplicated as a result of abnormal recanalization (most commonly near the ileocecal valve). The duplication is found on the mesenteric border; its lumen generally communicates with the normal bowel, shares the same blood supply as the normal bowel, and is lined by normal intestinal epithelium, but heterotopic gastric and pancreatic tissue has been identified. It is associated clinically with an abdominal mass, bouts of abdominal pain, vomiting, chronic rectal bleeding, intussusception, and perforation.

i. **Intussusception** occurs when a segment of bowel invaginates or telescopes into an adjacent bowel segment, leading to obstruction or ischemia. This is one of the most common causes of obstruction in children below 2 years of age, is most often idiopathic, and most commonly involves the ileum and colon (i.e., is ileocolic). It is associated clinically with intermittent abdominal pain of acute onset, vomiting, bloody stools, diarrhea, and somnolence.

j. **Retrocecal and retrocolic appendix** occurs when the appendix is located on the posterior side of the cecum or colon, respectively. These anomalies are very common and important to remember during appendectomies. Note: The appendix is normally found on the medial side of the cecum.

IV Hindgut Derivatives are supplied by the **inferior mesenteric artery (Figure 7-7).**

A. The distal third of the transverse colon, descending colon, sigmoid colon. The cranial end of the hindgut develops into the distal third of the transverse colon, descending colon, and sigmoid colon. The terminal end of the hindgut is an endoderm-lined pouch called the **cloaca,** which contacts the surface ectoderm of the **proctodeum** to form the **cloacal membrane.**

B. Rectum and upper anal canal

1. **Formation.** The cloaca is partitioned by the **urorectal septum** into the **rectum and upper anal canal** and the **urogenital sinus.** The cloacal membrane is partitioned by the urorectal septum into the **anal membrane** and **urogenital membrane.** Note: The urorectal septum fuses with the cloacal membrane at the future site of the gross anatomic **perineal body.**

2. **Clinical correlations**

   a. **Colonic aganglionosis (Hirschsprung disease)** is caused by the arrest of the caudal migration of neural crest cells. The hallmark is the absence of ganglionic cells in the myenteric and submucosal plexuses, most commonly in the sigmoid colon and rectum, resulting in a narrow segment of colon (i.e., the colon fails to relax). Although the ganglionic cells are absent, there is a proliferation of hypertrophied nerve fiber bundles. The most characteristic functional finding is failure of the internal anal sphincter to relax following rectal distention (i.e., abnormal rectoanal reflex). Mutations of the **RET proto-oncogene** (chromosome 10q.11.2) have been associated with Hirschsprung disease. This condition is associated clinically with a distended abdomen, inability to pass meconium, gushing of fecal material upon a rectal digital exam, and a loss of peristalsis in the colonic segment distal to the normal innervated colon.

   b. **Rectovesical, rectourethral, and rectovaginal fistulas** are abnormal communications between the rectum and urinary bladder (rectovesical), rectum and urethra (rectourethral), and rectum and vagina (rectovaginal) due to abnormal formation of the urorectal septum. These fistulas are associated clinically with the presence of meconium in the urine or vagina.

V The Anal Canal

A. Formation. The **upper anal canal** develops from the **hindgut.** The **lower anal canal** develops from the **proctodeum,** which is an invagination of surface ectoderm caused by a proliferation of mesoderm surrounding the anal membrane. The dual components (hindgut and proctodeum) involved in the embryological formation of the entire anal canal determine the gross anatomy of this area, which becomes important in considering the characteristics and metastasis of anorectal tumors. The junction between the upper and lower anal canals is indicated by the **pectinate line,** which also marks the site of the former **anal membrane.** In the adult, the pectinate line is located at the lower border of the anal columns.

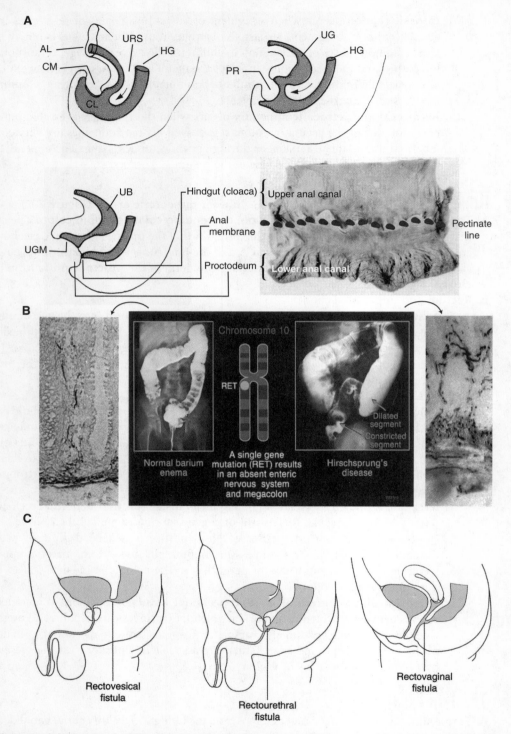

● **Figure 7.7 (A) Diagram depicting the partitioning of the cloaca (CL) by urorectal septum (URS).** CM = cloacal membrane, AL= allantois, HG = hindgut. The bold arrow shows the direction of growth of the urorectal septum. **(B) Hirschsprung disease.** Micrographs show nerve fibers stained for acetylcholinesterase. Note the proliferation of hypertrophied nerve fiber bundles in Hirschsprung disease. **(C) Rectovesical fistula, rectourethral fistula, and rectovaginal fistula.** A rectourethral fistula, which generally occurs in males, is associated with the prostatic urethra and is therefore sometimes called a rectoprostatic fistula.

B. Clinical correlations

1. **Imperforate anus** occurs when the anal membrane fails to perforate; a layer of tissue separates the anal canal from the exterior.

2. **Anal agenesis** occurs when the anal canal ends as a blind sac **below the puborectalis muscle** due to abnormal formation of the urorectal septum. It is usually associated with a rectovesical, rectourethral, or rectovaginal fistula.

3. **Anorectal agenesis** occurs when the rectum ends as a blind sac **above the puborectalis muscle** due to abnormal formation of the urorectal septum. It is the most common type of anorectal malformation and is usually associated with a rectovesical, rectourethral, or rectovaginal fistula.

4. **Rectal atresia** occurs when both the rectum and anal canal are present but remain unconnected due to either abnormal recanalization or a compromised blood supply, causing focal atresia.

 Mesenteries. The primitive gut tube is suspended within the peritoneal cavity of the embryo by a **ventral** and **dorsal mesentery,** from which all adult mesenteries are derived (Table 7-1).

TABLE 7-1	DERIVATION OF ADULT MESENTERIES
Embryonic Mesentery	**Adult Mesentery**
Ventral mesentery	Lesser omentum (hepatoduodenal and hepatogastric ligaments), falciform ligament, coronary ligament, and triangular ligament
Dorsal mesentery	Greater omentum (gastrorenal, gastrosplenic, gastrocolic, and splenorenal ligaments), mesentery of small intestine, mesoappendix, transverse meso colon, sigmoid mesocolon

Case Study 1

A 39-year-old man comes to your office complaining of "heartburn after trying to eat" and not being able to swallow anything. He states "I have tried everything from water to steaks. It doesn't matter what I eat; I always have trouble swallowing it down." What is the most likely diagnosis?

Differentials

• Neurological disorder, thyroid disease, thyroid mass, achalasia, infection, reflux esophagitis

Relevant Physical Exam Findings

• Dysphagia
• Normal thyroid upon palpation

Relevant Lab Findings

• Barium swallow x-ray shows a dilated esophagus with an area of distal stenosis. It looks almost like a "bird's beak."
• Normal thyroid levels.

Diagnosis

• Achalasia. The findings on the x-ray are a telltale sign of achalasia. Another telltale sign is that these patients have a dysphagia involving both solids and liquids. The physical and lab findings exclude thyroid disease and masses. Even though reflux esophagitis would present with heartburn, it is limited to dysphagia of solids only.

Case Study 2

A mother brings her 1-month-old son into the clinic complaining that her son is "vomiting all over the place when he tries to eat something." She says that her son's vomiting looks like it was "shot out of a cannon." What is the most likely diagnosis?

Differentials

- Hypertrophic pyloric stenosis, hiatal hernia, malrotation with volvulus

Relevant Physical Exam Findings

- Small, nontender, palpable mass on right costal margin

Relevant Lab Findings

- Barium swallow x-ray shows a narrow pyloric channel.
- Abdominal ultrasound shows a hypertrophic pylorus.

Diagnosis

- Hypertrophic pyloric stenosis

Case Study 3

A man brings his 3-year-old son into the office saying that the child has been having "bad stomach pains" as well as "running a fever" and "being thirsty all the time." The father remarks that his son has not had a bowel movement lately. What is the most likely diagnosis?

Differentials

- Volvulus, intussusception, indirect hernia, foreign body obstruction

Relevant Physical Exam Findings

- Painless rectal bleeding
- Abdominal distention

Relevant Lab Findings

- X-ray findings show a remnant of the vitelline duct, estimated to be about 2 ft from the ileocecal valve.
- No patent processus vaginalis is evident.
- Biopsy shows ectopic gastric and pancreatic mucosal tissue.

Diagnosis

- Meckel diverticulum. This condition occurs when a remnant of embryonic vitelline duct persists. It is associated with volvulus and intussusception. However, due to the finding of the remnants, these last two conditions can be excluded. No foreign body was found in the GI tract on x-ray. Also, an indirect hernia was ruled out because no patent processus vaginalis was detected, which is needed to make the diagnosis of an indirect hernia.

Case Study 4

A nurse comes into your office informing you that the child you delivered yesterday has failed to pass meconium. The nurse remarks that the child also cries when its abdominal area is palpated. What is the most likely diagnosis?

Differentials

- Hirschsprung disease, anal atresia, anal malformation, anal stenosis

Relevant Physical Exam Findings

- Abdominal distention
- Bilious vomiting
- Megacolon upon palpation

Relevant Lab Findings

- Barium enema shows a dilated proximal segment and a narrow distal segment.

Diagnosis

- Hirschsprung disease

Chapter 8

Urinary System

I **Overview** **(Figure 8-1).** The **intermediate mesoderm** forms a longitudinal elevation along the dorsal body wall called the **urogenital ridge.** A portion of the urogenital ridge forms the **nephrogenic cord,** which gives rise to the urinary system. The nephrogenic cord develops into three sets of nephric structures: the **pronephros, mesonephros,** and **metanephros.** The homeobox genes **Lim-1 and Pax-2** are important in the early stages of kidney development.

A. **The pronephros** develops by the differentiation of mesoderm within the nephrogenic cord to form **pronephric tubules** and the **pronephric duct.** The pronephros is the cranialmost nephric structure; it is a transitory structure that regresses completely by week 5. The pronephros is not functional in humans.

B. **The mesonephros** develops by the differentiation of mesoderm within the nephrogenic cord to form **mesonephric tubules** and the **mesonephric duct (Wolffian duct).** The mesonephros is the middle nephric structure and is partially transitory. Most of the mesonephric tubules regress, but the mesonephric duct persists and opens into the urogenital sinus. The mesonephros is functional for a short period.

C. **The metanephros** develops from an outgrowth of the mesonephric duct (called the **ureteric bud**) and from a condensation of mesoderm within the nephrogenic cord called the **metanephric mesoderm.** The metanephros is the caudalmost nephric structure. The metanephros begins to form at week 5 and is functional in the fetus at about week 10. The metanephros develops into the **definitive adult kidney.** The fetal kidney is divided into lobes, in contrast to the definitive adult kidney, which has a smooth contour.

II **Development of the Metanephros**

A. **Development of the collecting system.** The ureteric bud is an outgrowth of the mesonephric duct. This outgrowth is regulated by **WT-1** (an antioncogene), **GDNF** (glial cell line–derived neurotrophic factor), and **c-Ret** (a tyrosine kinase receptor). The ureteric bud initially penetrates the metanephric mesoderm and then undergoes repeated branching to form the **ureters, renal pelvis, major calyces, minor calyces,** and **collecting ducts.**

B. **Development of the nephron.** The inductive influence of the collecting ducts causes the metanephric mesoderm to differentiate into **metanephric vesicles,** which later give rise to primitive **S-shaped renal tubules; these** are critical to nephron formation. The S-shaped renal tubules differentiate into the **connecting tubule, distal convoluted tubule, loop of Henle, proximal convoluted tubule,** and **Bowman's capsule.** Tufts of capillaries called **glomeruli** protrude into Bowman's capsule. Nephron formation is complete at birth, but functional maturation of nephrons continues throughout infancy.

III **Relative Ascent of the Kidneys.** The fetal metanephros is located at vertebral level **S1-S2,** whereas the definitive adult kidney is located at vertebral level **T12-L3.** The change in location results from a disproportionate growth of the embryo caudal to the metanephros.

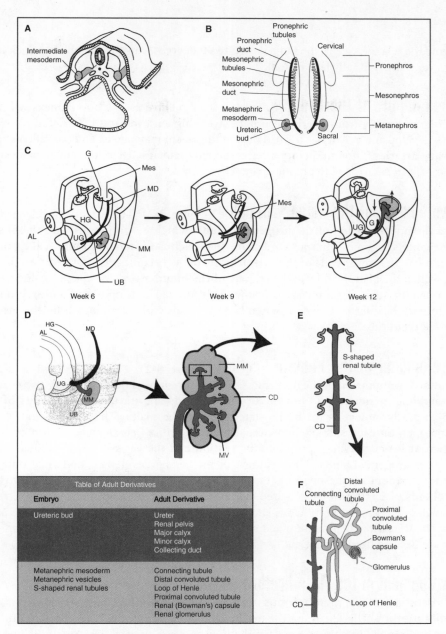

● Figure 8.1 (A) Cross-sectional view of an embryo at week 4. This figure illustrates the intermediate mesoderm as a cord of mesoderm that extends from the cervical to the sacral levels and forms the urogenital ridge and nephrogenic cord. **(B) Frontal view of an embryo, depicting the pronephros, mesonephros, and metanephros.** Note that nephric structures develop from cervical through sacral levels. **(C) Diagrams show the relationship between the gonad, mesonephros, and metanephros during development at weeks 6, 9, and 12.** Note that the gonad descends (arrow) while the metanephros ascends (arrow). G = gonad, Mes = mesonephros, MD = mesonephric duct, MM = metanephric mesoderm, HG = hindgut, AL = allantois, UB = ureteric bud, UG = urogenital sinus. **(D) Lateral view of the embryo, showing the relationship between the ureteric bud (UB; shaded), metanephric mesoderm (MM), and mesonephric duct (MD; black).** In addition, note the urogenital sinus (UG), hindgut (HD), and allantois (AL). Lateral view of a fetal kidney. Shaded area indicates structures formed from the ureteric bud. Note the repeated branching of the ureteric bud into the metanephric mesoderm (MM). At the tip of each collecting duct (CD), the formation of metanephric vesicles (MV) is induced. Note the lobulated appearance of a fetal kidney. MI = minor calyx, MJ = major calyx, P = pelvis, U = ureter. **(E) Enlarged view of the rectangle shown in D, illustrating the further branching of a collecting duct (CD; shaded) and the formation of primitive S-shaped renal tubules.** **(F) Diagram showing a collecting duct (CD) and the six components of a mature adult nephron.** A summary table of derivatives is shown.

During the relative ascent, the kidneys **rotate 90 degrees,** causing the hilum, which initially faces ventrally, to finally face medially.

(IV) **Blood Supply of the Kidneys.** During their relative ascent, the kidneys will receive their blood supply from arteries at progressively higher levels until the definitive renal arteries develop at **L2.** Arteries formed during the ascent may persist and are called **supernumerary arteries.** Supernumerary arteries are **end arteries.** Therefore any damage to them will result in necrosis of the kidney parenchyma.

(V) **Development of the Urinary Bladder** (Figure 8-2). The urinary bladder is formed from the upper portion of the **urogenital sinus,** which is continuous with the **allantois.** The allantois becomes a fibrous cord called the **urachus** (or **median umbilical ligament** in the adult). The lower ends of the mesonephric ducts become incorporated into the posterior wall of the bladder to form the **trigone of the bladder.** The mesonephric ducts eventually open into the urogenital sinus below the bladder. The **transitional epithelium** lining the urinary bladder is derived from endoderm because of its etiology from the urogenital sinus and gut tube.

(VI) **Development of the Female Urethra** (Figure 8-2). The female urethra is formed from the lower portion of the urogenital sinus. It develops endodermal outgrowths into the surrounding mesoderm to form the **urethral glands** and **paraurethral glands of Skene** (which are homologous to the prostate gland in the male). The paraurethral glands of Skene open on each side of the external urethral orifice. The female urethra ends at the **navicular fossa,** which empties into the **vestibule of the vagina;** this vestibule also forms from the urogenital sinus. The vestibule of the vagina develops endodermal outgrowths into the surrounding mesoderm to form the **lesser vestibular glands** and **greater vestibular glands of Bartholin** (which are homologous to the bulbourethral glands of Cowper in the male). The greater vestibular glands of Bartholin open on each side of the vaginal orifice. The transitional epithelium and stratified squamous epithelium lining the female urethra are derived from endoderm.

(VII) **Development of the Male Urethra** (Figure 8-2)
A. **Prostatic urethra, membranous urethra, bulbous urethra, and proximal part of penile urethra.** These parts of the urethra are formed from the lower portion of the urogenital sinus. The transitional epithelium and stratified columnar epithelium lining these parts of the urethra are derived from endoderm.
   1. **The prostatic urethra** develops endodermal outgrowths into the surrounding mesoderm to form the **prostate gland.** The posterior wall of the prostatic urethra has an elevation called the urethral crest. The prostatic sinus is a groove on either side of the urethral crest that receives most of the prostatic ducts from the prostate gland. At a specific site along the urethral crest, there is an ovoid enlargement called the **seminal colliculus** (also called the **verumontanum**), which contains the **openings of the ejaculatory ducts** and the **prostatic utricle** (a vestigial remnant of the paramesonephric ducts in the male, which is involved in the development of the vagina and uterus).
   2. **The membranous urethra** develops endodermal outgrowths into the surrounding mesoderm to form the **bulbourethral glands of Cowper.**
   3. **The bulbous urethra** contains the openings of the bulbourethral glands of Cowper.

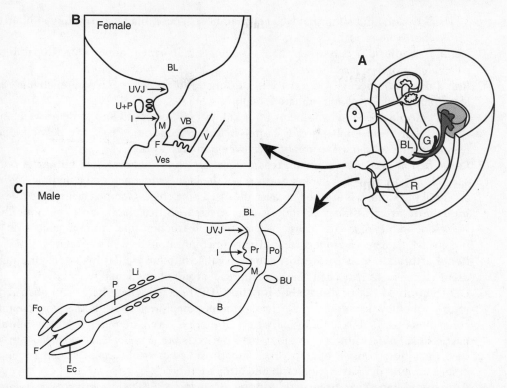

● **Figure 8.2 (A) Diagram of an embryo, showing the development of the upper portion of the urogenital sinus into the urinary bladder (BL) and the lower portion into the female and male urethra. (B) Female urethra.** The bladder (BL), membranous portion of the female urethra (M), and navicular fossa (F) are shown; they empty into the vestibule of the vagina (Ves). In addition, the urethrovesical junction (UVJ) and intermuscular incisura (I) are shown. U + P = urethral and paraurethral glands of Skene, VB = lesser and greater vestibular glands of Bartholin, V = vagina. **(C) Male urethra.** The bladder (BL), prostatic urethra (Pr), membranous urethra (M), bulbous urethra (B), proximal part of the penile urethra (P), and navicular fossa (F) are shown. In addition, the urethrovesical junction (UVJ) and intermuscular incisura (I) are shown. Pr = prostate gland, BU = bulbourethral glands of Cowper, Li = urethral glands of Littré, Fo = foreskin, Ec = ectodermal septa.

4. **The proximal part of the penile urethra** develops endodermal outgrowths into the surrounding mesoderm to form the **urethral glands of Littré.**

B. **The distal part of the penile urethra** is formed from an ingrowth of surface ectoderm called the **glandular plate.** The glandular plate joins the proximal penile urethra and becomes canalized to form the **navicular fossa. Ectodermal septa** appear lateral to the navicular fossa and become canalized to form the **foreskin.** The stratified squamous epithelial lining of the distal penile urethra is derived from ectoderm.

 Clinical Correlations (Figure 8-3)

A. **Renal agenesis** occurs when the ureteric bud fails to develop, thereby eliminating the induction of metanephric vesicles and nephron formation.

1. **Unilateral renal agenesis** is relatively common (more common in males). Therefore a physician should never assume that a patient has two kidneys. This condition is asymptomatic and compatible with life, because the remaining kidney hypertrophies.

2. **Bilateral renal agenesis** is relatively uncommon. It causes oligohydramnios, which causes compression of the fetus and hence **Potter syndrome** (deformed limbs,

wrinkly skin, and abnormal facial appearance). These infants are usually stillborn or die shortly after birth.

B. **Renal hypoplasia** occurs when there is a congenitally small kidney with no pathological evidence of dysplasia.

C. **Renal dysplasia** occurs when there is a disorganization of the renal parenchyma, with abnormally developed and immature nephrons.

D. **Renal ectopia** occurs when one or both kidneys fail to ascend and therefore remain in the pelvis or lower lumbar area (i.e., **pelvic kidney**). In some cases, two pelvic kidneys fuse to form a solid mass, commonly called a **pancake kidney.**

E. **Renal fusion.** The most common type of renal fusion is the **horseshoe kidney.** A horseshoe kidney occurs when the inferior poles of the kidneys fuse across the midline. Normal ascent of the kidneys is arrested because the fused portion gets trapped behind the **inferior mesenteric artery.** Kidney rotation is also arrested, so that the hilum faces ventrally. A horseshoe kidney may also cause urinary tract obstruction due to impingement on the ureters, which may lead to recurrent urinary tract infections as well as pyelonephritis.

F. **Renal artery stenosis** is the most common cause of renovascular hypertension in children. The stenosis may occur in the main renal artery of segmental renal arteries.

G. **Obstruction of the ureteropelvic junction (UPJ)** occurs when there is an obstruction to the urine flow from the renal pelvis to the proximal ureter. UPJ is the most common congenital obstruction of the urinary tract. If there is severe uteropelvic atresia, a **multicystic dysplastic kidney** is found, where the cysts are actually dilated calyces. In this case, the kidney consists of grape-like, smooth-walled cysts of variable size. Between the cysts are found dysplastic glomeruli and atrophic tubules.

H. **Autosomal recessive polycystic kidney disease** (**ARPKD;** formerly called infantile polycystic kidney disease) is an autosomal recessive disease that has been mapped to the short arm of chromosome 6 (p6). In ARPKD, the kidneys (always bilateral) are huge and spongy, with a smooth external surface; they contain numerous cysts due to the dilatation of collecting ducts and tubules, which severely compromises kidney function. ARPKD is associated clinically with cysts of the liver, pancreas, and lungs as well as with hepatic fibrosis (hepatic hypertension). Treatment includes dialysis and kidney transplant. In contrast, **autosomal dominant polycystic kidney disease** (**ADPKD;** formerly called adult polycystic disease) is an autosomal dominant disease that has been mapped to chromosome 16. In ADPKD, the kidneys are bilaterally enlarged, with a distorted external surface due to the protrusion of cysts; they contain numerous large cysts (up to 5 cm in diameter) that arise anywhere along the nephrons and are filled with a straw-colored fluid. The cysts are not present at birth but develop over time, so that renal function is retained until 30–40 years of age. ADPKD is associated clinically with hypertension, abdominal pain, hematuria, renal stones, cysts of the liver and pancreas, diverticulosis, intracranial berry aneurysms, and mitral valve prolapse.

I. **Wilms tumor (WT).** WT is the **most common renal malignancy of childhood.** WT is the most common primary tumor of childhood and is typically due to a deletion of

tumor suppressor gene WT1, located on chromosome 11. WT presents as a large, solitary, well-circumscribed mass that, on cut section, is soft, homogeneous, and tan-gray in color. WT is interesting histologically in that this tumor tends to recapitulate different stages of embryological formation of the kidney, so that three classic histological areas are described: a stromal area, a blastemal area of tightly packed embryonic cells, and a tubular area. WT can be associated with hemihypertrophy (asymmetrical unilateral muscular hypertrophy). WT is associated with other congential anomalies called the WAGR complex [**W**ilms tumor, **a**niridia (absence of the iris), **g**enitourinary malformations, and mental **r**etardation].

J. **Ureteropelvic duplications** occur when the ureteric bud divides prematurely, before penetrating the metanephric blastema. This results in either a double kidney or duplicated ureter and renal pelvis. The term "duplex kidney" refers to a configuration where two ureters drain one kidney.

K. **Exstrophy of the bladder** occurs when the posterior wall of the urinary bladder is exposed to the exterior. It is caused by a failure of the anterior abdominal wall and anterior wall of the bladder to develop properly. It is associated clinically with urinary drainage to the exterior and epispadias. Surgical reconstruction is difficult and prolonged.

L. **Urachal fistula or cyst** occurs when a remnant of the allantois persists, thereby forming fistula or cyst. It is found along the midline on a path from the umbilicus to the apex of the urinary bladder. A urachal fistula forms a direct connection between the urinary bladder and the outside of the body at the umbilicus, causing **urinary drainage** from the umbilicus.

M. **Ectopic opening of the ureter** occurs when the ureteric bud fails to separate from the mesonephric duct, which results in the opening of the ureter being carried to a point distal to its normal position. The most common ectopic opening is a **lateral ureteral ectopia,** where the opening is lateral to its normal position.

   1. **In males,** the ectopic openings are most commonly located in the prostatic urethra, ejaculatory ducts, ductus deferens, or rectum. Because the ectopic openings are all located above the external urethral sphincter, boys with an ectopic opening of the ureter do not present with urinary incontinence.

   2. **In females,** the ectopic openings are most commonly located in the urethra, vestibule, or vagina. Because the ectopic openings are all located below the external urethral sphincter, girls with an ectopic opening of the ureter generally present with urinary incontinence.

N. **Ureterocele**

   1. **Simple ureterocele** occurs when the distal end of the ureter has a cyst-like protrusion into the submucosal layer of the urinary bladder.

   2. **Ectopic ureterocele** occurs when the distal end of the ureter has a cyst-like protrusion into the submucosal layer of the urinary bladder; this is almost invariably associated with an ectopic ureter and duplication. In this situation, the ureterocele is at the end of the ureter from the upper renal segment and is located inferior to the other ureter opening.

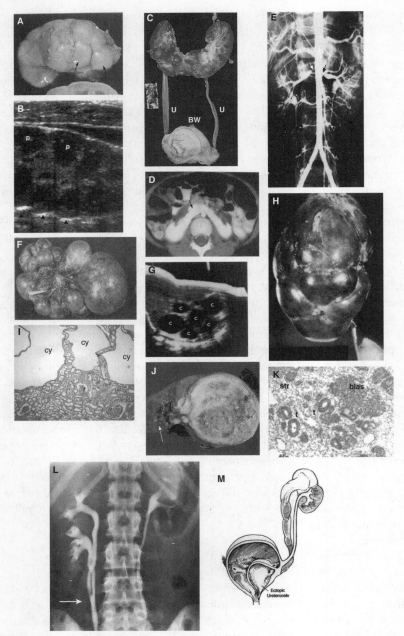

● **Figure 8.3 (A,B) Normal newborn kidney.** Photograph shows the normal lobation pattern (arrows). Sonogram shows mounds (arrowheads) indicating the fetal lobes. The renal pyramids (p) are less echoic than the surrounding renal cortex. **(C,D) Horseshoe kidney.** Photograph of a horseshoe kidney. U = ureter, BW = bladder wall. CT shows the isthmus of renal tissue (arrow) that extends across the midline. **(E) Renal artery stenosis.** Angiogram shows bilateral renal artery stenosis (arrows). **(F,G) Multidysplastic kidney.** Photograph shows numerous cysts. Sonogram shows many anechoic cysts (c) separated by renal septa. **(H,I) Autosomal recessive polycystic kidney disease (ARPKD).** Photograph of a polycystic kidney. LM shows large, fluid-filled cysts (cy) usually confined to the collecting ducts and tubules. Between the cysts, some functioning nephrons can be observed. **(J,K) Wilms tumor.** Photograph shows the Wilms tumor extending from normal kidney tissue (arrow). LM shows the tumor, which is characterized histologically by recognizable attempts to recapitulate embryonic development of the kidney. In this regard, the following three components are seen: (a) metanephric blastema elements (blas) consisting of clumps of small, tightly packed embryonic cells; (b) stromal elements (str); and (c) epithelial elements, generally in the form of abortive attempts at forming tubules (t) or glomeruli. **(L) Ureteropelvic duplication.** The intravenous urogram (IVU) shows duplication of the collecting system on the right side. The two ureters fuse at vertebral level L4 (arrow). However, they may remain separate throughout their course and open separately. The ureter from the lower pole opens normally at the urinary bladder trigone. However, the ureter from the upper pole usually has an ectopic opening. **(M) Ectopic ureterocele**. The ureterocele is shown at the end of an enlarged ureter from the upper renal segment. The opening of the enlarged ureter is located inferior to the normal-sized ureter from the lower renal segment.

IX   Development of the Suprarenal Gland (Figure 8-4)

A. Cortex. The cortex forms from two episodes of mesodermal proliferation that occur between the root of the dorsal mesentery and the gonad. The first episode forms the inner **fetal cortex.** The second episode forms the outer **adult cortex,** whereby mesodermal proliferation occurs at the periphery of the fetal cortex. During the fetal period and at birth, the suprarenal glands are very large, due to the size of the fetal cortex. The suprarenal glands become smaller as the fetal cortex involutes rapidly during the first 2 weeks after birth and continues to involute during the first year of life. The zona glomerulosa and zona fasciculata of the adult cortex are present at birth, but the zona reticularis is not formed until age 3 years.

B. Medulla. The medulla forms when neural crest cells aggregate at the medial aspect of the fetal cortex and eventually become surrounded by the fetal and adult cortex. The neural crest cells differentiate into **chromaffin cells,** which stain yellow-brown with chromium salts. Chromaffin cells can be found in extrasuprarenal sites at birth, but these sites will normally regress completely by puberty. In a normal adult, chromaffin cells are found only in the suprarenal medulla.

C. Clinical considerations

1. **Neuroblastoma (NB).** NB is a common extracranial malignant neoplasm containing **primitive neuroblasts** (small cells arranged in **Homer-Wright pseudorosettes**) of **neural crest origin.** NB results from an amplification of the **N-*myc* oncogene,** which is a nuclear transcription factor involved in cell proliferation. NB occurs mainly in children and is found in extra-adrenal sites, usually along the sympathetic chain ganglia (60%) or within the adrenal medulla (40%). NB metastasizes widely to the bone marrow, bone, and lymph nodes. A common laboratory finding is increased levels of urine vanillylmandelic acid (VMA) and metanephrine.

2. **Pheochromocytoma (PH).** PH is a relatively rare, mainly benign neoplasm that contains both epinephrine and norepinephrine. PH occurs mainly in adults 40–60 years of age and is generally found in the region of the adrenal gland but may be found in extra suprarenal sites. PH is associated with persistent or paroxysmal hypertension, anxiety, tremor, profuse sweating, pallor, chest pain, and abdominal pain. Laboratory findings include increased levels of urinary VMA and metanephrine, inability to suppress catecholamines with clonidine, and hyperglycemia. PH may be associated with von Hippel-Lindau disease or neurofibromatosis. PH is treated by surgery or phenoxybenzamine (an α-adrenergic antagonist).

3. **Congenital adrenal hyperplasia (CAH).** CAH is caused most commonly by mutations in genes for enzymes involved in adrenocortical steroid biosynthesis (e.g., **21-hydroxylase deficiency, 11β-hydroxylase deficiency**). In 21-hydroxylase deficiency (90% of all cases), there is virtually no synthesis of cortisol or aldosterone, so that intermediates are funneled into androgen biosynthesis, thereby elevating androgen levels. The elevated levels of androgens lead to **masculinization of a female fetus** (i.e., **female pseudointersexuality**). This condition produces the following clinical findings: mild clitoral enlargement, complete labioscrotal fusion with a phalloid organ, or macrogenitosomia (in the male fetus). Since cortisol cannot be synthesized, negative feedback to the adenohypophysis does not occur; therefore adrenocorticotropic hormone (ACTH) continues to stimulate the adrenal cortex, resulting in adrenal hyperplasia. Since aldosterone cannot be synthesized, the patient presents with **hyponatremia ("salt-wasting")** with associated **dehydration** and **hyperkalemia.** Treatment includes immediate infusion of intravenous saline and long-term steroid hormone replacement, both cortisol and mineralocorticoids (9α-fludrocortisone).

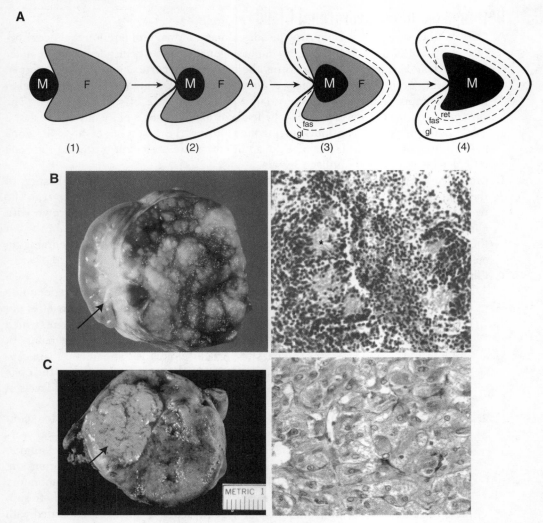

● **Figure 8.4 (A) Development of the suprarenal gland.** (1) At week 6, the fetal cortex (F) and medulla (M) at the medial aspect of the adrenal gland are apparent. (2) At week 9, the adult cortex (A) has formed at the periphery of the fetal cortex. Note that the medulla is completely surrounded by the adult and fetal cortex. (3) At birth, the fetal cortex is still present and the adult cortex has differentiated into the zona glomerulosa (gl) and zona fasciculata (fas). (4) At 3 years of age, the fetal cortex has completely involuted, thus reducing the size of the suprarenal gland, and the adult cortex has further differentiated to form the zona reticularis (ret). **(B) Neuroblastoma.** Neuroblastomas vary in size from 1 cm to filling the entire abdomen. They are generally soft and white to gray-pink in color. As the size increases, the tumors become hemorrhagic, also undergoing calcification and cyst formation. Note the nodular appearance of this tumor, with the kidney apparent on its left border (arrow). LM shows that the neoplastic cells are small, primitive-looking cells with dark nuclei and scant cytoplasm. The cells are generally arranged as solid sheets, and some cells are arranged around a central fibrillar area, forming Homer-Wright pseudorosettes (∗). **(C) Pheochromocytoma.** Pheochromocytomas vary from 3–5 cm in diameter. They are gray-white to pink-tan in color. Exposure of the cut surface often results in darkening of the surface due to the formation of yellow-brown adenochrome pigment. This pheochromocytoma shows a prominent area of fibrosis (arrow). LM shows neoplastic cells that have abundant cytoplasm with small centrally located nuclei. The cells are generally grouped into clusters separated by a slender stroma and numerous capillaries. Many cytoplasmic hyaline eosinophilic globules are sometimes present, which are derived from membranes of secretory granules.

Case Study 1

A 33-year-old man comes into the clinic complaining of "fever and chills" and that he "is constantly going to the bathroom." He also indicates that he has pain in the right lower abdomen. He states he has not had sex in more than 6 months. He suspects that the problem may be a urinary tract infection because he "has had a lot of them over the years." What is the most likely diagnosis?

Differentials

- UTI (urinary tract infection), pyelonephritis, kidney stones

Relevant Physical Exam Findings

- Flank pain
- Costovertebral angle (CVA) tenderness

Relevant Lab Findings

- Normal calcium levels
- Presence of leukocytes
- Horseshoe kidney present on CT scan

Diagnosis

- Horseshoe kidney. The symptoms reported by the patient (fevers, chills, flank pain, and CVA tenderness) are classic signs of pyelonephritis as a result of a UTI. In this case, the UTI is due to urinary tract obstruction caused by a horseshoe kidney.

Case Study 2

A parent brings his 4-year-old daughter into the clinic. He says he has noticed "a lump" on his daughter's lower right side that has "gotten bigger over time." What is the most likely diagnosis?

Differentials

- Unilateral renal agenesis, neuroblastoma, Wilms tumor

Relevant Physical Exam Findings

- Large palpable mass on the right flank
- Kidney size normal

Relevant Lab Findings

- No UTI
- No increase in catecholamine
- No increase in androgen production
- Genetic testing reveals deletion of the tumor suppression gene on chromosome 11

Diagnosis

- Wilms tumor. This is the most common primary renal tumor in childhood; it normally presents as a large palpable flank mass with hemihypertrophy. Unilateral renal agenesis is ruled out because, although the patient would have renal hypertrophy on one side, she would also have only one kidney. Neuroblastoma is ruled out because there was no mention of an increase in levels of urinary VMA and metanephrine.

Case Study 3

A 45-year-old man comes into the clinic complaining of chest and abdominal pain. He also says that his "blood pressure was rising every so often" when he was not exercising and that "it's been happening more and more." He says he works out often and tries to stay in shape because he has a family history of obesity. What is the most likely diagnosis?

Differentials

- Myocardial infarction, acute renal failure, angina, pulmonary embolism, pneumothorax, pheochromocytoma

Relevant Physical Exam Findings

- Profuse sweating
- Hypertension
- Abdominal discomfort
- Lungs clear on auscultation

Relevant Lab Findings

- Chest x-ray is negative for pulmonary embolism
- Increased urinary VMA
- Increased metanephrine levels
- Inability to suppress catecholamines with clonidine; hyperglycemia

Diagnosis

- Pheochromocytosis. Lab findings for pheochromocytoma include an increase in urinary VMA and metanephrine levels, inability to suppress catecholamines with clonidine, and hyperglycemia.

Chapter 9

Female Reproductive System

I The Indifferent Embryo. The genotype of the embryo (46,XX or 46,XY) is established at fertilization. **During weeks 1–6,** the embryo remains in a sexually indifferent or undifferentiated stage. This means that genetically female embryos and genetically male embryos are phenotypically indistinguishable. **During week 7,** the indifferent embryo begins phenotypic sexual differentiation. **By week 12,** female or male characteristics of the external genitalia can be recognized. **By week 20,** phenotypic differentiation is complete.

A. Phenotypic sexual differentiation is determined by the *Sry* **gene** located on the short arm of the Y chromosome and may result in individuals with a **female phenotype,** an **intersex phenotype,** or a **male phenotype.** The *Sry* gene encodes for a protein called **testes-determining factor (TDF).** TDF is 220-amino acid nonhistone protein that contains a highly conserved DNA-binding region called a **high-mobility group box.** As the indifferent gonad develops into the testes, Leydig cells and Sertoli cells differentiate to produce **testosterone** and **MIF (müllerian inhibiting factor),** respectively. In the presence of TDF, testosterone, and MIF, the indifferent embryo will be directed to the male phenotype. In the absence of TDF, testosterone, and MIF, the indifferent embryo will be directed to the female phenotype.

B. The components of the indifferent embryo that are remodeled to form the adult female reproductive system include the **gonads, genital ducts,** and **primordia of external genitalia.** Phenotypic sexual differentiation occurs in a sequence beginning with the gonads, then the genital ducts, and finally with the primordia of external genitalia.

II Development of the Gonads

A. **The ovary.** The **intermediate mesoderm** forms a longitudinal elevation along the dorsal body wall, the **urogenital ridge.** The coelomic epithelium and underlying mesoderm of the urogenital ridge proliferate to form the **gonadal ridge. Primary sex cords** develop from the gonadal ridge and incorporate primordial germ cells (XX genotype), which migrate into the gonad from the wall of the yolk sac. Primary sex cords extend into the medulla and develop into the **rete ovarii,** which eventually degenerates. Later, **secondary sex cords** develop and incorporate primordial germ cells as a thin **tunica albuginea** forms. The secondary sex cords break apart and form isolated cell clusters called **primordial follicles,** which contain **primary oocytes** surrounded by a layer of **simple squamous cells.** Primary oocytes, simple squamous cells, and connective tissue stroma of the ovary are derived from mesoderm.

B. **Relative descent of the ovaries.** The ovaries originally develop within the abdomen but later undergo a relative descent into the pelvis as a result of disproportionate growth of the upper abdominal region away from the pelvic region. Other factors in this movement are uncertain but probably include the **gubernaculum.** The gubernaculum is a band of fibrous tissue along the posterior wall that extends from the medial pole of the ovary to the uterus at the junction of the uterine tubes, forming the **ovarian ligament.** The gubernaculum then continues into the labia majora, forming the **round ligament of the uterus.** The peritoneum evaginates alongside the gubernaculum to form the **processus vaginalis,** which is obliterated in the female later in development.

III ## Development of the Genital Ducts (Figure 9-1)

A. **Paramesonephric (müllerian) ducts** develop as invaginations of the lateral surface of the urogenital ridge. The cranial portions develop into the **uterine tubes.** The caudal portions fuse in the midline to form the **uterovaginal primordium** and thereby bring together two peritoneal folds called the **broad ligament.** The uterovaginal primordium develops into the **uterus, cervix,** and **superior third of the vagina.** The paramesonephric ducts project into the dorsal wall of the cloaca and induce the formation of the **sinovaginal bulbs.** The sinovaginal bulbs fuse to form the solid **vaginal plate,** which canalizes and develops into the **inferior two-thirds of the vagina.** Although the vagina has a dual origin, most authorities agree that the epithelial lining of the entire vagina is of endodermal origin. Vestigial remnants of the paramesonephric duct may be found in the adult female and are called the **hydatid of Morgagni.**

B. **Mesonephric (wolffian) ducts and tubules** develop in the female as part of the urinary system, since these ducts are critical in the formation of the definitive metanephric kidney. However, they degenerate in the female after formation of the metanephric kidney. Vestigial remnants of the mesonephric ducts, called the **appendix vesiculosa** and **Gartner's duct,** may be found in the adult female. Vestigial remnants of the mesonephric tubules, called the **epoophoron** and **paroophoron,** may be found in the adult female.

IV ## Development of the Primordia of External Genitalia (Figure 9-2) A proliferation of mesoderm around the cloacal membrane causes the overlying ectoderm to rise up, so that three structures are visible externally; these include the **phallus, urogenital folds,** and **labioscrotal swellings.** The phallus forms the **clitoris (glans clitoris, corpora cavernosa clitoris,** and **vestibular bulbs).** The urogenital folds form the **labia minora.** The labioscrotal swellings form the **labia majora** and **mons pubis.**

V ## Clinical Considerations

A. **Uterine anomalies (Figure 9-3)**

1. **Müllerian hypoplasia or agenesis anomalies (class I)** involving the paramesonephric ducts can result in vaginal, cervical, uterine, uterine tube, or combined anomalies.

2. **Unicornuate uterus anomalies (class II)** occur when one paramesonephric duct fails to develop or develops incompletely.

3. **Didelphys (double uterus) anomalies (class III)** occur when there is a complete lack of fusion of the paramesonephric ducts.

4. **Bicornuate uterus anomalies (class IV)** occur when there is partial fusion of the paramesonephric ducts.

5. **Septate uterus anomalies (class V)** occur when the medial walls of the caudal portion of the paramesonephric ducts fail to resorb partially or completely.

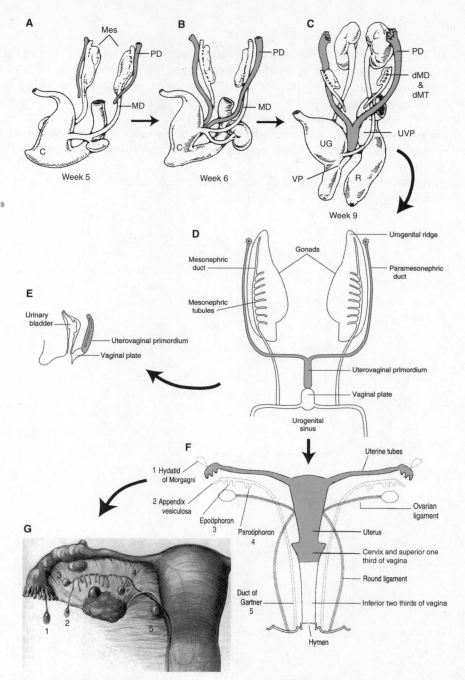

● **Figure 9.1 (A–C) Lateral view of the embryo. (A)** At week 5: Paired paramesonephric ducts (PD) begin to form along the lateral surface of the urogenital ridge at the mesonephros (Mes) and grow in close association to the mesonephric duct (MD). **(B)** At week 6: The paramesonephric ducts (PD) grow caudally and project into the dorsal wall of the cloaca (C) and induce the formation of the sinovaginal bulbs (not shown). The mesonephric ducts (MD) continue to prosper. **(C)** At week 9: The caudal portions of the paramesonephric ducts (PD) fuse in the midline to form the uterovaginal primordium (UVP) and the sinovaginal bulbs fuse to form the vaginal plate (VP) at the urogenital sinus (UG). During this time, the mesonephric duct and mesonephric tubules both degenerate in the female (dMD and dMT). R = rectum. **(D) Genital ducts in the indifferent embryo. (E) Lateral view showing the dual origin of the vagina. (F) Female components and vestigial remnants (dotted lines) at birth. (G) Location of various cysts that are encountered clinically within the female reproductive tract.** The formation of cysts is related to vestigial remnants of the genital ducts. 1 = Kobelt's cyst arises from the appendix vesiculosa, which is a remnant of the mesonephric duct, 2 = cyst of the epoophoron (type II) arises from the epoophoron, which is a remnant of the mesonephric tubules, 3 = cyst of the paroophoron arises from the paroophoron, which is a remnant of the mesonephric tubules, 4 = Gartner's duct cyst, which arises from the duct of Gartner, a remnant of the mesonephric duct, 5 = hydatid cyst of Morgagni, which arises from hydatid of Morgagni, a remnant of the paramesonephric duct.

6. **DES-related anomalies.** Diethylstilbestrol (DES) was used until 1970 in the treatment of abortions, preeclampsia, diabetes, and preterm labor. For female offspring (i.e., daughters) exposed to DES in utero, an increased incidence of vaginal and cervical adenocarcinoma has been documented. In addition, many uterine anomalies, including a T-shaped uterus, have been observed.

B. **Hymen variations** include **crescentic hymen, annular hymen, redundant hymen, imperforate hymen, cribriform hymen, microperforate hymen, and septate hymen.**

C. **Atresia of the vagina** is a condition where the vaginal lumen is blocked due to a failure of the vaginal plate to canalize and form a lumen.

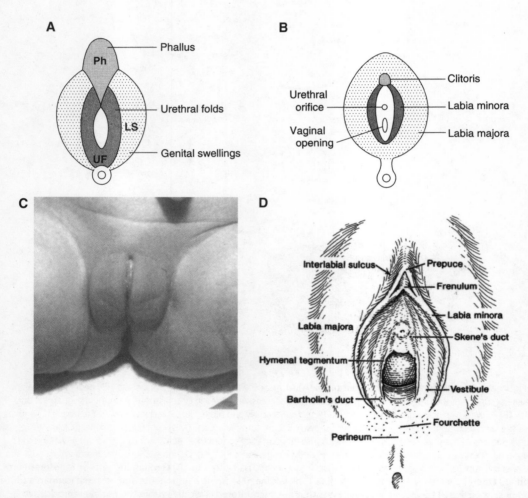

● Figure 9.2 **(A,B)** Diagrams indicating the differentiation of the phallus (Ph), urogenital folds (UF), and labioscrotal swellings (LS) in the female. **(A)** At week 5. **(B)** At birth. **(C)** Appearance of normal female genitalia at birth. **(D)** Diagram of the gross anatomy of the vulvar region in the adult female.

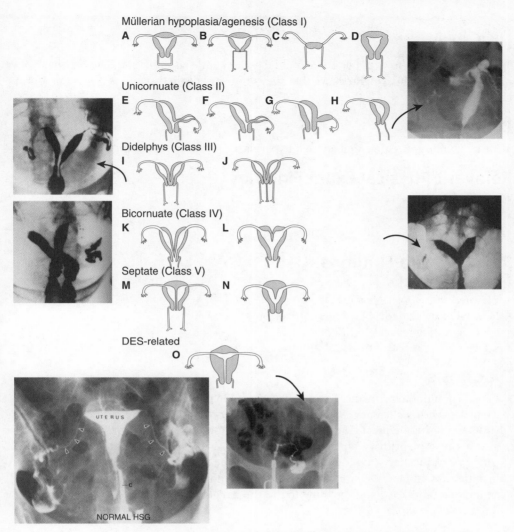

● **Figure 9.3 Diagram depicting various congenital anomalies of the uterus and vagina. (A–D)** Müllerian hypoplasia and agenesis anomalies, Class I: **(A)** Lower vaginal agenesis. **(B)** Cervical agenesis. **(C)** Uterine and cervical hypoplasia. **(D)** Uterine tube agenesis. **(E–H)** Unicornuate anomalies, Class II: **(E)** Unicornuate uterus with a communicating rudimentary horn. **(F)** Unicornuate uterus with a noncommunicating rudimentary horn. **(G)** Unicornuate uterus with a rudimentary horn containing no uterine cavity. **(H)** Unicornuate uterus. Hysterosalpingography (HSG) shows a single lenticular uterine canal with no evidence of a rudimentary right horn. There is filling of the left uterine tube. **(I,J)** Didelphys (double uterus) anomalies, class III: **(I)** Didelphys with normal vagina. An HSG shows a double uterus with a single normal vagina (top panel). **(J)** Didelphys with complete vaginal septum. An HSG shows a double uterus with a double vagina due to vaginal septum (bottom panel). This 17-year-old girl uses two tampons during menses. **(K,L)** Bicornuate anomalies, Class IV: **(K)** Bicornuate uterus with complete division down to the internal os. **(L)** Bicornuate uterus with partial division. An HSG shows the uterine cavity partitioned into two channels. **(M,N)** Septate uterine anomalies, Class V: **(M)** Septate uterus with complete septum down to the external os. **(N)** Septate uterus with partial septum. **(O)** DES-related uterine anomalies. These anomalies typically result in a T-shaped uterus. An HSG shows a T-shaped uterus. An HSG of a normal female reproductive tract is shown for comparison. Arrowheads = uterine tubes, c = catheter in the cervical canal.

Case Study

A woman comes in with her 16-year-old daughter and states that her daughter has not yet had a menstrual. The daughter says that she is not sexually active and is not on any form of birth control.

Differentials

- Turner syndrome, congenital adrenal hyperplasia, pituitary tumor, pituitary insufficiency

Relevant Physical Exam Findings

- Ambiguous genitalia
- Amenorrhea
- Early appearance of axillary and pubic hair

Relevant Lab Findings

- Elevated urinary 17-ketosteroids
- Elevated serum DHEA sulfate
- Normal or decreased 17-hydroxycorticosteroids
- Genetic testing reveals 46,XX genotype
- CT head scan reveals no sign of tumor

Diagnosis

- Female pseudointersexuality (congenital adrenal hyperplasia) occurs when a woman has a 21-hydroxylase deficiency, which prevents the formation of aldosterone and cortisol and shifts the hormone precursors to form male sex hormones. Although Turner syndrome is also a cause of primary amenorrhea, individuals with Turner syndrome have a 45,XO genotype. A pituitary tumor can be excluded by the negative CT scan findings. A pituitary insufficiency can be ruled out because adrenal gland hormone production is present, indicating that pituitary gland signaling to the adrenal glands is intact.

Chapter 10

Male Reproductive System

I **The Indifferent Embryo.** The genotype of the embryo (46,XX or 46,XY) is established at fertilization. **During weeks 1–6,** the embryo remains in a sexually indifferent or undifferentiated stage. This means that genetically female embryos and genetically male embryos are phenotypically indistinguishable. **During week 7,** the indifferent embryo begins phenotypic sexual differentiation. **By week 12,** female or male characteristics of the external genitalia can be recognized. **By week 20,** phenotypic differentiation is complete.

A. Phenotypic sexual differentiation is determined by the *Sry* **gene,** located on the short arm of the Y chromosome, and may result in individuals with a **female phenotype,** an **intersex phenotype,** or a **male phenotype.** The *Sry* gene encodes for a protein called **testes-determining factor (TDF).** TDF is 220-amino acid nonhistone protein that contains a highly conserved DNA-binding region called a **high-mobility-group box.** As the indifferent gonad develops into the testes, Leydig cells and Sertoli cells differentiate to produce **testosterone** and **MIF (müllerian inhibiting factor),** respectively. In the presence of TDF, testosterone, and MIF, the indifferent embryo will be directed to the male phenotype. In the absence of TDF, testosterone, and MIF, the indifferent embryo will be directed to the female phenotype.

B. The components of the indifferent embryo that are remodeled to form the adult female reproductive system include the **gonads, genital ducts,** and **primordia of external genitalia.** Phenotypic sexual differentiation occurs in a sequence beginning with the gonads, then the genital ducts, and finally with the primordia of external genitalia.

II **Development of the Gonads**

A. The testes. The **intermediate mesoderm** forms a longitudinal elevation along the dorsal body wall, the **urogenital ridge.** The coelomic epithelium and underlying mesoderm of the urogenital ridge proliferate to form the **gonadal ridge. Primary sex cords** develop from the gonadal ridge and incorporate primordial germ cells (XY genotype), which migrate into the gonad from the wall of the yolk sac. The Y chromosome carries a gene on its short arm that codes for **testes-determining factor (TDF),** which is crucial to testes differentiation. The primary sex cords extend into the medulla of the gonad and lose their connection with the surface epithelium as the thick **tunica albuginea** forms. The primary sex cords form the **seminiferous cords, tubuli recti,** and **rete testes.** Seminiferous cords consist of **primordial germ cells** and **sustentacular (Sertoli) cells,** which secrete **müllerian-inhibiting factor (MIF).** The mesoderm between the seminiferous cords gives rise to the **interstitial (Leydig) cells,** which secrete **testosterone.** The primordial germ cells, sustentacular (Sertoli) cells, interstitial (Leydig) cells, and connective tissue stroma of the testes are derived from mesoderm. The seminiferous cords remain as solid cords until puberty, when they acquire a lumen and are then called **seminiferous tubules.**

B. Relative descent of the testes. The testes originally develop within the abdomen but later undergo a relative descent into the scrotum as a result of disproportionate growth of the upper abdominal region away from the pelvic region. Other factors involved in this movement are uncertain but probably include the **gubernaculum.** The gubernaculum is a band of fibrous tissue along the posterior wall that extends from the caudal pole of the testes to the scrotum. Remnants of the gubernaculum in the adult male serve to anchor the testes within the scrotum. The peritoneum evaginates alongside the gubernaculum to form the **processus vaginalis.** Later in development, most of the processus vaginalis is obliterated except at its distal end, which remains as a peritoneal sac called the **tunica vaginalis** of the testes.

III Development of the Genital Ducts (Figure 10-1)

A. Paramesonephric (müllerian) ducts develop as invaginations of the lateral surface of the urogenital ridge. The cranial portions run parallel to the mesonephric ducts. The caudal portions fuse in the midline to form the uterovaginal primordium. Under the influence of MIF, the cranial portions of the paramesonephric ducts and the uterovaginal primordium regress. Vestigial remnants of the paramesonephric duct (called the **appendix testis**) may be found in the adult male.

B. Mesonephric (wolffian) ducts and tubules develop in the male as part of the urinary system, since these ducts are critical in the formation of the definitive metanephric kidney. The mesonephric ducts then proceed to additionally form the **epididymis, ductus deferens, seminal vesicle,** and **ejaculatory duct.** A few mesonephric tubules in the region of the testes form the **efferent ductules** of the testes. Vestigial remnants of the mesonephric duct (called the **appendix epididymis**) and the mesonephric tubules (called the **paradidymis**) may be found in the adult male.

IV Development of the Primordia of External Genetalia (Figure 10-2). A proliferation of

mesoderm around the cloacal membrane causes the overlying ectoderm to rise up, so that three structures are visible externally; these include the **phallus, urogenital folds,** and **labioscrotal swellings.** The phallus forms the **penis (glans penis, corpora cavernosa penis, and corpus spongiosum penis).** The urogenital folds form the **ventral aspect of the penis (i.e., penile raphe).** The labioscrotal swellings form the **scrotum.**

V Clinical Considerations

A. Male anomalies (Figure 10-3)

1. **Hypospadias** occurs when the urethral folds fail to fuse completely, so that the external urethral orifice opens onto the ventral surface of the penis. It is generally associated with a poorly developed penis that curves ventrally, known as **chordee.**

2. **Epispadias** occurs when the external urethral orifice opens onto the dorsal surface of the penis. It is generally associated with **exstrophy of the bladder.**

3. **Undescended testes (cryptorchidism)** occurs when the testes fail to descend into the scrotum. Descent of the testes is evident within 3 months of birth. Bilateral cryptorchidism results in **sterility.** The undescended testes may be found in the abdominal cavity or in the inguinal canal.

4. **Hydrocele of the testes** occurs when a small patency of the processus vaginalis remains, so that peritoneal fluid can flow into the processus vaginalis. This results in a fluid-filled cyst near the testes, seen as a scrotal enlargement that transilluminates due to persistence of the tunica vaginalis.

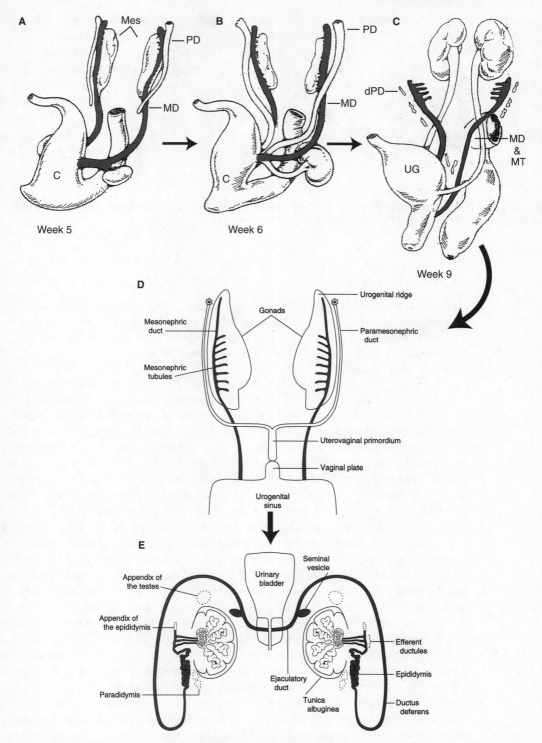

● **Figure 10.1 (A–C) Lateral view of the embryo. (A)** At week 5: Paired paramesonephric ducts (PD) begin to form along the lateral surface of the urogenital ridge at the mesonephros (Mes) and grow in close association to the mesonephric duct (MD). **(B)** At week 6: The paramesonephric ducts (PD) grow caudally and project into the dorsal wall of the cloaca (C) and induce the formation of the sinovaginal bulbs (not shown). The mesonephric ducts (MD) continue to prosper. **(C)** At week 9: The mesonephric ducts (MD) and mesonephric tubules establish contact with the testes and develop into definitive adult structures. During this period, the paramesonephric ducts degenerate in the male (dPD). **(D) Genital ducts in the indifferent embryo. (E) Male components and vestigial remnants (dotted lines).** The mesonephric ducts/tubules and their derivatives are shaded.

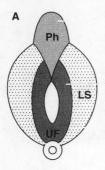

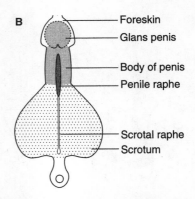

● **Figure 10.2 (A,B) Diagrams indicating the differentiation of the phallus (Ph), urogenital folds (UF), and labioscrotal swellings (LS) in the male. (A)** At week 5. **(B)** At birth.

5. **Congenital inguinal hernia** occurs when a large patency of the processus vaginalis remains, so that a loop of intestine may herniate into the scrotum or labia majora. It is most common in males and is generally associated with cryptorchidism.

B. **Other anomalies of the reproductive system (Figure 10-4)**

1. **Intersexuality.** Because the early embryo goes through an indifferent stage, events may occur whereby a fetus does not progress toward either of the two usual phenotypes but gets caught in an intermediate stage known as intersexuality. Intersexuality is classified according to the histologic appearance of the **gonad** and **ambiguous genitalia. True intersexuality** occurs when an individual has both ovarian and testicular tissue (ovotestes) histologically, ambiguous genitalia, and a 46,XX genotype. True intersexuality is a rare condition whose cause is poorly understood.

2. **Female pseudointersexuality (FP)** occurs when an individual has only ovarian tissue histologically and masculinization of the female external genitalia. These individuals have a **46,XX genotype.** FP is most often observed clinically in association with a condition in which the fetus produces an **excess of androgens [e.g., congenital adrenal hyperplasia (CAH)].** CAH is caused most commonly by mutations in genes for enzymes involved in adrenocortical steroid biosynthesis (e.g., **21-hydroxylase deficiency, 11β-hydroxylase deficiency**). **In 21-hydroxylase deficiency (90% of all cases),** there is virtually no synthesis of cortisol or aldosterone, so that intermediates are funneled into androgen biosynthesis, thereby elevating androgen levels. The elevated levels of androgens lead to **masculinization of a female fetus.** FP produces the following clinical findings: mild clitoral enlargement, complete labioscrotal fusion with a phalloid organ, or macrogenitosomia (in the male fetus). Since cortisol cannot be synthesized, negative feedback to the adenohypophysis does not occur, so that adrenocorticotropic hormone (ACTH) continues to stimulate the adrenal cortex, resulting in adrenal hyperplasia. Since aldosterone cannot be synthesized, the patient presents with **hyponatremia ("salt wasting"),** with associated **dehydration** and **hyperkalemia.** Treatment includes immediate infusion of intravenous saline and long-term steroid hormone replacement, both cortisol and mineralocorticoids (9α-fludrocortisone).

3. **Male pseudointersexuality (MP)** occurs when an individual has only testicular tissue histologically and various stages of stunted development of the male external genitalia. These individuals have a **46,XY genotype.** MP is most often observed clinically in association with a condition in which the fetus produces a **lack of**

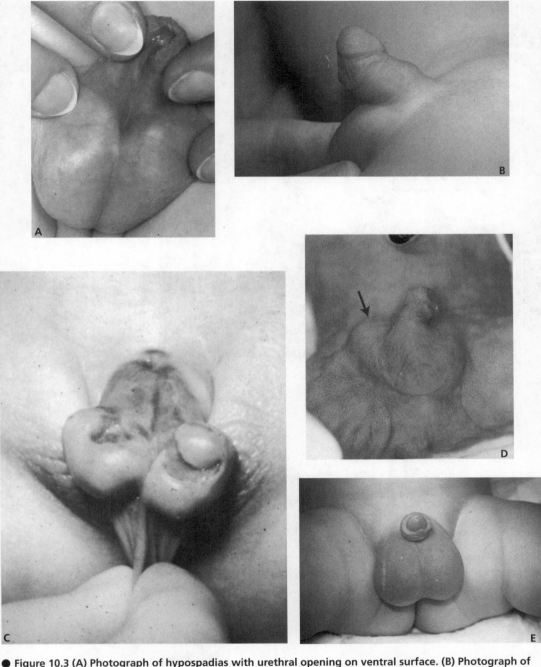

● Figure 10.3 (A) Photograph of hypospadias with urethral opening on ventral surface. (B) Photograph of chordee. Note that the penis is poorly developed and bowed ventrally. (C) Photograph of epispadias with the urethral opening on the dorsal surface of the penis, whereby the penis is almost split in half. (D) Photograph of cryptorchidism. Note that neither testis has descended into the scrotal sac. (E) Photograph of bilateral hydrocele.

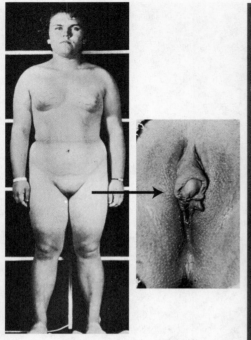

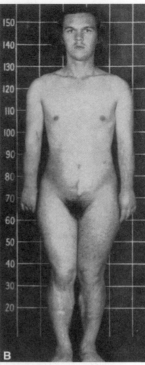

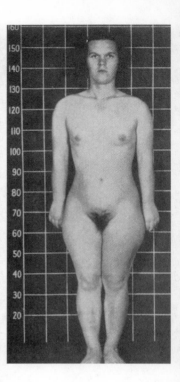

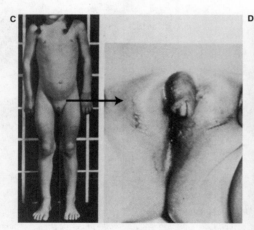

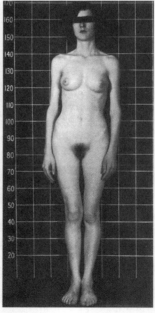

● **Figure 10.4 (A) A patient (XX genotype) with female pseudointersexuality due to congenital adrenal hyperplasia.** Masculinization of female external genitalia is apparent, with fusion of the labia majora and enlarged clitoris (see arrow to inset). **(B) A patient (XX genotype) with female pseudointersexuality due to congenital adrenal hyperplasia (i.e., 21-hydroxylase deficiency).** This 10-year-old girl is clearly masculinized (left panel). After 9 months of cortisone therapy, there is marked improvement (right panel). **(C) A patient (XY genotype) with male pseudointersexuality.** Stunted development of male external genitalia is apparent. The stunted external genitalia fooled parents and physician into thinking that this XY infant was a girl. In fact, this child was raised as a girl (note pigtails). As this child neared puberty, testosterone levels increased and clitoral enlargement ensued. This alarmed the parents and the child was brought in for clinical evaluation. **(D) A patient (XY genotype) with complete androgen insensitivity (CAIS or testicular feminization).** Complete feminization of male external genitalia is apparent.

androgens (and MIF). This is caused most commonly by mutations in genes for androgen steroid biosynthesis (e.g., **5α-reductase 2 deficiency** or **17β-hydroxy-steroid dehydrogenase**). Normally, 5α-reductase 2 catalyzes the conversion of testosterone → dihydrotestosterone and 17β HSD 3 catalyzes the conversion of androstenedione → testosterone. An increased **T:DHT ratio** is diagnostic (normal = 5; 5α-reductase 2 deficiency = 20–60). The reduced levels of androgens lead to the **feminization of a male fetus.** MP produces the following clinical findings: underdevelopment of the penis, and scrotum (microphallus, hypospadias, and bifid scrotum), and prostate gland. The epididymis, ductus deferens, seminal vesicle, and ejaculatory duct are normal. These clinical findings have led to the inference that DHT is essential in the development of the penis and scrotum (external genitalia) and prostate gland in the genotypic XY fetus. At puberty, these individuals demonstrate a striking virilization.

4. **Complete androgen insensitivity (CAIS) or testicular feminization syndrome** occurs when a fetus with a 46,XY genotype develops testes and female external genitalia with a rudimentary vagina; uterus and uterine tubes are generally absent. The testes may be found in the labia majora and are surgically removed to circumvent malignant tumor formation. These individuals present as normal-appearing females, and their psychosocial orientation is female despite their genotype. The most common cause is a mutation in the gene for the **androgen receptor.** Even though the developing male fetus is exposed to normal levels of androgens, the lack of androgen receptors renders the phallus, urogenital folds, and labioscrotal swellings unresponsive to androgens.

Ⓥ Summary Table of Female and Male Reproductive System Development (Table 10-1)

TABLE 10-1	DEVELOPMENT OF THE MALE AND FEMALE REPRODUCTIVE SYSTEMS	
Adult Female	**Indifferent Embryo**	**Adult Male***
Ovary, ovarian follicles, rete ovarii	**Gonads**	Testes, seminiferous tubules, tubuli recti, rete testes, Leydig cells, Sertoli cells
Uterine tubes, uterus, cervix, superior third of vagina, *hydatid of Morgagni*	**Paramesonephric duct**	*Appendix testes*
Appendix vesiculosa, Gartner's duct*	**Mesonephric duct**	Epididymis, ductus deferens, seminal vesicle, ejaculatory duct, *appendix epididymis*
Epoophoron, paroophoron	**Mesonephric tubules**	Efferent ductules, *paradidymis*
Glans clitoris, corpora cavernosa clitoris, vestibular bulbs	**Phallus**	Glans penis, corpora cavernosa penis, corpus spongiosum
Labia minora	**Urogenital folds**	Ventral aspect of penis
Labia majora, mons pubis	**Labioscrotal swellings**	Scrotum
Ovarian ligament, round ligament of uterus	**Gubernaculum**	Gubernaculum testes
	Processus vaginalis	Tunica vaginalis

* Italics indicate vestigial structures.

Case Study

A concerned couple brings their 3-week-old son into your office stating that they think something is wrong with their son's genitals. They noticed that his testicles appeared to be swollen when they were changing his diaper a week earlier and that his scrotum felt like a "water-filled balloon." Neither parent could recall any traumatic episode with their son, saying that they have been very protective of him.

Differentials

- Hydrocele, hematocele, inguinal hernia, obstruction within spermatic cord

Relevant Physical Exam Findings

- Enlarged scrotum that is nontender
- Testicles not immediately palpable
- No herniated bulge found
- Flashlight test through the enlarged area showed illumination

Relevant Lab Findings

- Negative for blood on fluid collection
- Ultrasound confirmation of hydrocele

Diagnosis

- Hydrocele occurs when there is a patent tunica vaginalis. Peritoneal fluid drains from the abdomen through the tunica vaginalis. The fluid accumulates in the scrotum, becomes trapped, and causes the scrotum to enlarge. A hydrocele is usually harmless and in most cases resolves within a few months after birth. A hydrocele is normally treated only when there is discomfort or when the testicular blood supply is threatened. A hematocele could have also been considered, but a hematocele is typically due to trauma, and blood would have been seen on fluid collection. Inguinal hernias usually accompany hydroceles, but no bulge was detected on physical examination. Obstruction within the spermatic cord is usually seen in older men.

Chapter 11

Respiratory System

I **The Upper Respiratory System** consists of the **nose, nasopharynx,** and **oropharynx.**

II **The Lower Respiratory System** (**Figure 11-1**) consists of the **larynx, trachea, bronchi,** and **lungs.** The first sign of development is the formation of the **respiratory diverticulum** in the ventral wall of the primitive foregut during week 4. The distal end of the respiratory diverticulum enlarges to form the **lung bud.** The lung bud divides into two **bronchial buds, which** branch into the **main (primary), lobar (secondary), segmental (tertiary), and subsegmental bronchi.** The respiratory diverticulum initially is in open communication with the foregut, but eventually they become separated by indentations of mesoderm, the **tracheoesophageal folds.** When the tracheoesophageal folds fuse in the midline to form the **tracheoesophageal septum,** the foregut is divided into the trachea ventrally and esophagus dorsally.

A. **Development of the larynx.** The opening of the respiratory diverticulum into the foregut becomes the **laryngeal orifice.** The laryngeal epithelium and glands are derived from endoderm. The laryngeal muscles are derived from somitomeric mesoderm of pharyngeal arches 4 and 6 and therefore are innervated by branches of the vagus nerve (CN X); i.e., the superior laryngeal nerve and recurrent laryngeal nerve, respectively. The laryngeal cartilages (thyroid, cricoid, arytenoid, corniculate, and cuneiform) are derived from somitomeric mesoderm of pharyngeal arches 4 and 6.

B. **Development of the trachea. Clinical correlation. Tracheoesophageal fistula** is an abnormal communication between the trachea and esophagus due to improper division of foregut by the tracheoesophageal septum. It is generally associated with **esophageal atresia** and **polyhydramnios.** Clinical features include excessive accumulation of saliva or mucus in the nose and mouth, episodes of gagging and cyanosis after swallowing milk, abdominal distention after crying, and reflux of gastric contents into lungs, causing pneumonitis. Diagnostic features include inability to pass a catheter into the stomach and radiographs demonstrating air in the stomach.

C. **Development of the bronchi (Figure 11-2)**

1. **Stages of development.** The lung bud divides into two bronchial buds. In week 5 of development, the bronchial buds enlarge to form the **main (primary) bronchi.** The right main bronchus is larger and more vertical than the left main bronchus; this relationship persists throughout adult life and accounts for the greater likelihood of foreign bodies lodging on the right side than on the left. The main bronchi further subdivide into **lobar (secondary) bronchi** (3 on the right side and 2 on the left, corresponding to the lobes of the adult lung). The lobar bronchi further subdivide into **segmental (tertiary) bronchi** (10 on the right side and 9 on the left) which further subdivide into **subsegmental bronchi.** The segmental bronchi are the primordia of the **bronchopulmonary segments,** which are morphologically and functionally separate

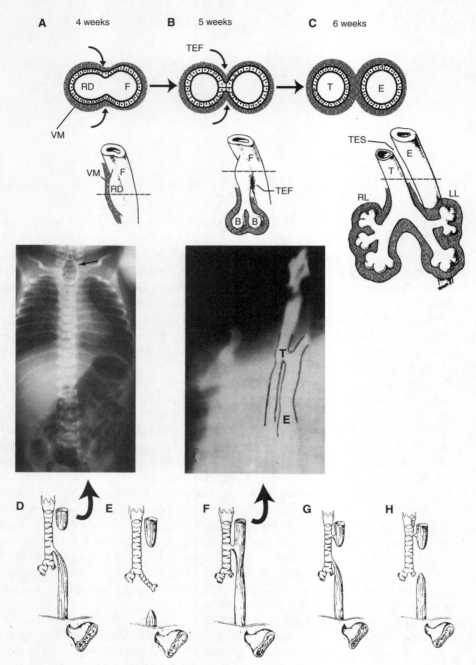

● **Figure 11.1 Development of the respiratory system at (A) 4 weeks, (B) 5 weeks, and (C) 6 weeks.**
Both lateral views and cross-sectional views are shown. Note the relationship of the respiratory diverticulum (RD) and foregut (F). Curved arrows indicate the movement of the tracheoesophageal folds (TEF) as the tracheoesophageal septum (TES) forms between the trachea (T) and esophagus (E). B = bronchial buds, RL = right lung, LL = left lung. **(D–H) Five different anatomic types of esophagus and tracheal malformations. (D)** Esophageal atresia with a tracheoesophageal fistula at the distal third (end) of the trachea. This is the most common type, occurring in 82% of cases. The AP radiograph of this malformation shows an enteric tube (arrow) coiled in the upper esophageal pouch. The air in the bowel indicates a distal tracheoesophageal fistula. **(E)** Esophageal atresia only, occurring in 9% of the cases. **(F)** H-type tracheoesophageal fistula only, occurring in 6% of the cases. The barium swallow radiograph shows a normal esophagus (E), but dye has spilled into the trachea (T) through the fistula and outlines the upper trachea and larynx. **(G)** Esophageal atresia with a tracheoesophageal fistula at both proximal and distal ends, occurring in 2% of the cases. **(H)** Esophageal atresia with a tracheoesophageal fistula at the proximal end, occurring in 1% of the cases.

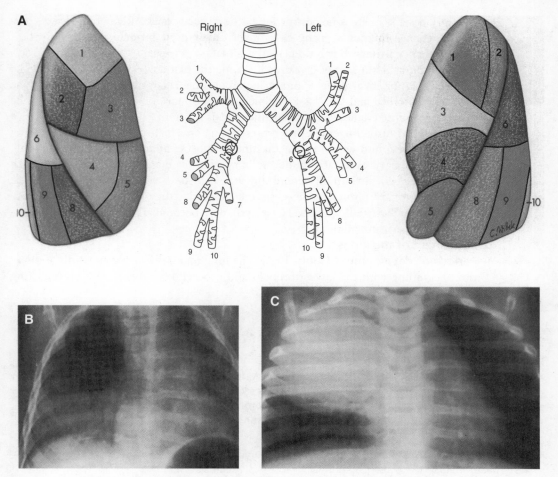

● **Figure 11.2 (A) Distribution of bronchopulmonary segments and their relationship to the tracheo-bronchial tree.** Segmental bronchi of the right and left lungs are numbered. Right lung: 1, 2, and 3, segmental bronchi that branch from the upper lobar bronchus; 4, and 5, segmental bronchi that branch from the middle lobar bronchus; 6, 7, 8, 9, and 10: segmental bronchi that branch from the lower lobar bronchus. Note that bronchopulmonary segment, no. 7, is not represented on the outer costal surface of the right lung (no. 7 is located on the inner mediastinal surface). Left lung: 1, 2, 3, 4, and 5, segmental bronchi that branch from the upper lobar bronchus; 6, 8, 9, and 10, segmental bronchi that branch from the lower lobar bronchus. Note that there is no no. 7 segmental bronchus associated with the left lung. **(B) Congenital lobar emphysema.** Expiratory AP radiograph shows a hyperlucent area in the emphysematous right upper lobe due to air trapping. **(C) Congenital bronchogenic cyst.** AP radiograph shows a large opaque area in the right upper lobe due to a fluid-filled cyst.

respiratory units of the lung. As the bronchi develop, they expand laterally and caudally into a space known as the primitive pleural cavity. The visceral mesoderm covering the outside of the bronchi develops into **visceral pleura,** and somatic mesoderm covering the inside of the body wall develops into **parietal pleura.** The space between the visceral and parietal pleurae is called the **pleural cavity.**

2. **Clinical correlations**
   a. **The bronchopulmonary segment** is a segment of lung tissue supplied by a segmental (tertiary) bronchus. Surgeons can resect diseased lung tissue along bronchopulmonary segments rather than removing the entire lobe.
   b. **Congenital lobar emphysema (CLE)** is characterized by progressive overdistention of one of the upper lobes or the right middle lobe with **air.** The term "emphysema" is

a misnomer, as there is no destruction of the alveolar walls. Although the exact etiology remains unknown, many cases involve **collapsed bronchi** due to **failure of bronchial cartilage formation.** In this situation, air can be inspired through collapsed bronchi but cannot be expired. During the first few days of life, fluid may be trapped in the involved lobe, producing an opaque, enlarged hemithorax. Later, the fluid is resorbed and the classic radiological appearance of an emphysematous lobe with generalized radiolucency (hyperlucency) is apparent.

    c. **Congenital bronchogenic cysts** represent an abnormality in bronchial branching and may be found within the mediastinum (most commonly) or within the lung. Intrapulmonary cysts are round, solitary, sharply marginated, and **filled with fluid;** they do not initially communicate with the tracheobronchial tree. Since intrapulmonary bronchogenic cysts contain fluid, they appear as water-density masses on chest radiographs. These cysts may become air-filled as a result of infection or instrumentation.

D. Development of the lungs

   1. Periods of development (Table 11-1). The lung matures in a proximal-distal direction, beginning with the largest bronchi and proceeding outward. As a result, lung

TABLE 11-1	PERIODS OF DEVELOPMENT

Pseudoglandular period (weeks 7–16)
- The developing lung resembles an exocrine gland whereby numerous **endodermal tubules** are lined by a **simple columnar epithelium** and are surrounded by mesoderm containing a **modest capillary network**
- Each endodermal tubule branches into 15–20 **terminal bronchioles.**
- **Respiration is not possible and premature infants cannot survive.**

Canalicular period (weeks 16–24)
- The terminal bronchioles branch into 3 or more **respiratory bronchioles.**
- The respiratory bronchioles subsequently branch into 3–6 **alveolar ducts.**
- The terminal bronchioles, respiratory bronchioles, and alveolar ducts are now lined by a **simple cuboidal epithelium** and are surrounded by mesoderm containing a **prominent capillary network.**
- **Premature infants born before week 20 rarely survive.**

Terminal sac period (week 24–birth)
- The alveolar ducts bud off **terminal sacs,** which dilate and expand into the surrounding mesoderm.
- The terminal sacs are separated from each other by **primary septa.**
- The simple cuboidal epithelium within the terminal sacs differentiates into **type I pneumocytes** (thin, flat cells that make up part of the blood-air barrier) and **type II pneumocytes** (which secrete surfactant).
- The terminal sacs are surrounded by mesoderm containing a **rapidly proliferating capillary network.** The capillaries make intimate contact with the terminal sacs and thereby establish a **blood-air barrier** with the type I pneumocytes.
- **Premature infants born between weeks 25 and 28 can survive with intensive care.** Adequate vascularization and surfactant levels are the most important factors for the survival of premature infants.

Alveolar period (week 32 to 8 years of age)
- The terminal sacs are partitioned by **secondary septa** to form adult **alveoli.** About 20–70 million alveoli are present at birth. About 300–400 million alveoli are present by 8 years of age.
- The major mechanism for the increase in the number of alveoli is formation of secondary septa that partition existing alveoli.
- After birth, the increase in the size of the lung is due to an increase **in the number of respiratory bronchioles.**
- On chest radiographs, lungs of a newborn infant are denser than an adult lung because of the fewer number of mature alveoli.

development is heterogeneous; proximal pulmonary tissue will be in a more advanced period of development than distal pulmonary tissue. The periods of lung development include the **pseudoglandular period (weeks 7–16), canalicular period (weeks 16–24), terminal sac period (week 24 to birth), and alveolar period (week 32 to age 8 years).**

2. **Clinical correlations**
   a. **Aeration at birth** is the replacement of lung liquid with air in the newborn's lungs. In the fetal state, the functional residual capacity (FRC) of the lung is filled with liquid secreted by fetal lung epithelium via Cl^- transport using CFTR (cystic fibrosis transmembrane protein). At birth, lung liquid is eliminated by a reduction in the secretion of lung liquid via Na^+ transport by type II pneumocytes and resorption into pulmonary capillaries (major route) and lymphatics (minor route). Lungs of a stillborn baby will sink when placed in water because they contain fluid rather than air.
   b. **Pulmonary agenesis** is the complete absence of a lung or a lobe and its bronchi. This is a rare condition caused by failure of bronchial buds to develop. Unilateral pulmonary agenesis is compatible with life.
   c. **Pulmonary aplasia** is the absence of lung tissue but the presence of a rudimentary bronchus.
   d. **Pulmonary hypoplasia (PH)** is a poorly developed bronchial tree with abnormal histology. PH classically involves the right lung in association with right-sided obstructive congenital heart defects. PH can also be found in association with **congenital diaphragmatic hernia** (i.e., herniation of abdominal contents into the thorax), which compresses the developing lung. PH can also be found in association with **bilateral renal agenesis,** which causes an insufficient amount of amniotic fluid (oligohydramnios) to be produced; this, in turn, increases pressure on the fetal thorax.
   e. **Respiratory distress syndrome** (RDS; Figure 11-3) is caused by a deficiency or absence of **surfactant.** This surface-active agent is composed of **cholesterol** (50%), **dipalmitoylphosphatidylcholine** (DPPC; 40%), and **surfactant proteins A, B, and C** (10%); it coats the inside of alveoli to maintain alveolar patency. RDS is prevalent in premature infants (it accounts for 50%–70% of deaths in premature infants), infants of diabetic mothers, infants who experienced fetal asphyxia or maternofetal hemorrhage (damages type II pneumocytes), and multiple-birth infants. Clinical signs include dyspnea, tachypnea, inspiratory retractions of the chest wall, expiratory grunting, cyanosis, and nasal flaring. Treatments include administration of betamethasone (a corticosteroid) to the mother for several days before delivery (i.e., antenatally) to increase surfactant production, postnatal administration of an artificial surfactant solution, and postnatal high-frequency ventilation. RDS in premature infants cannot be discussed without mentioning **germinal matrix hemorrhage (GMS).** The germinal matrix is the site of proliferation of neuronal and glial precursors in the developing brain; it is located above the caudate nucleus, in the floor of the lateral ventricles, and the caudothalamic groove. The germinal matrix also contains a rich network of fragile, thin-walled blood vessels. The brain of the premature infant lacks the ability to autoregulate the cerebral blood pressure. Consequently, increased arterial blood pressure in these blood vessels causes rupture and hemorrhage into the germinal matrix. This leads to significant neurologic sequelae, including cerebral palsy, mental retardation, and seizures. Antenatal corticosteroid administration has a clear role in reducing the incidence of GMH in premature infants.

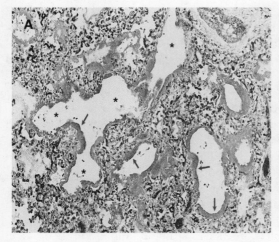
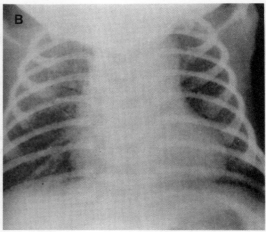

● **Figure 11.3 Respiratory distress syndrome (RDS). (A)** Light micrograph. The pathological hallmarks are acinar atelectasis (i.e., collapse of the respiratory acinus, which includes the respiratory bronchioles, alveolar ducts, and alveoli), dilation of terminal bronchioles (*), and deposition of an eosinophilic hyaline membrane material (arrows) consisting of fibrin and necrotic cells. **(B)** AP radiograph. The radiological hallmarks are a bell-shaped thorax due to underaeration and reticulogranularity of the lungs caused by acinar atelectasis.

Case Study

A mother brings her 5-year-old son into your office on a follow-up visit. The child previously had a bout of pneumonia and the mother says that he has been coughing up "yellow and green stuff." The mother remarks that he has had a number of coughs and colds that were just like this in the past. His chart indicates that he has cystic fibrosis. What is the most likely diagnosis?

Differentials

• Asthma, bronchitis, pneumonia

Relevant Physical Exam Findings

• Foul-smelling greenish sputum with speckles of blood
• Orthopnea
• Fever

Relevant Lab Findings

• Spirometry shows a reduced FEV_1/FVC ratio
• Chest x-ray shows multiple cysts that have a "honeycomb" appearance
• CT shows dilation of bronchi

Diagnosis

• Bronchiectasis

Chapter 12

Head and Neck

I **The Pharyngeal Apparatus** (**Figure 12-1**) consists of the **pharyngeal arches, pharyngeal pouches, pharyngeal grooves,** and **pharyngeal membranes,** all of which contribute greatly to the formation of the head and neck. The pharyngeal apparatus is first observed in week 4 of development and gives the embryo its distinctive appearance. There are five pharyngeal arches (1, 2, 3, 4, and 6), four pharyngeal pouches (1, 2, 3, and 4), four pharyngeal grooves (1, 2, 3, and 4), and four pharyngeal membranes (1, 2, 3, and 4). Pharyngeal arch 5 and pharyngeal pouch 5 completely regress in the human. Aortic arch 5 also completely regresses (see Chapter 5). The **Hox complex** and **retinoic acid** appear to be important factors in early head and neck formation. A lack or excess of retinoic acid causes striking facial anomalies.

A. **Pharyngeal arches (1, 2, 3, 4, and 6)*** contain **somitomeric mesoderm** and **neural crest cells.** In general, the mesoderm differentiates into **muscles** and **arteries** (i.e., aortic arches 1–6); whereas neural crest cells differentiate into **bone** and **connective tissue.** In addition, each pharyngeal arch has a **cranial nerve** associated with it.

B. **Pharyngeal pouches (1, 2, 3, and 4)** are evaginations of endoderm that lines the foregut.

C. **Pharyngeal grooves (1, 2, 3, and 4)** are invaginations of ectoderm located between each pharyngeal arch.

D. **Pharyngeal membranes (1, 2, 3, and 4)** are structures consisting of ectoderm, intervening mesoderm and neural crest, and endoderm located between each pharyngeal arch.

II **Development of the Thyroid Gland.** In the midline of the floor of the pharynx, the endodermal lining of the foregut forms the **thyroid diverticulum.** The thyroid diverticulum migrates caudally, passing ventral to the hyoid bone and laryngeal cartilages. During this migration, the thyroid remains connected to the tongue by the **thyroglossal duct,** which is later obliterated. The site of the thyroglossal duct is indicated in the adult by the **foramen cecum.**

III **Development of the Tongue** (**Figure 12-2A**)

A. **The oral part (anterior two-thirds) of the tongue** forms from the **median tongue bud** and **two distal tongue buds,** which develop in the floor of the pharynx associated with **pharyngeal arch 1.** The distal tongue buds overgrow the median tongue bud and fuse in the midline, forming the **median sulcus.** The oral part is characterized by **filiform papillae** (no taste buds), **fungiform papillae** (taste buds present), **foliate papillae** (taste buds present), and **circumvallate papillae** (taste buds present). General sensation from the mucosa is carried by the **lingual branch of the trigeminal nerve (CN V).** Taste sensation from the mucosa is carried by the **chorda tympani branch of the facial nerve (CN VII).**

---

* = pharyngeal arch 5 regresses in humans.

85

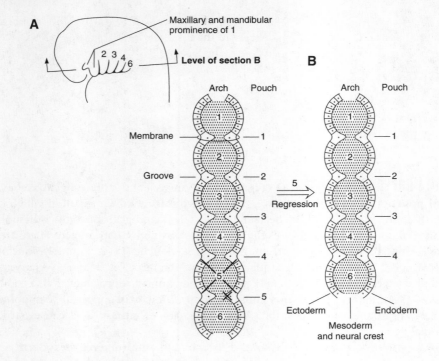

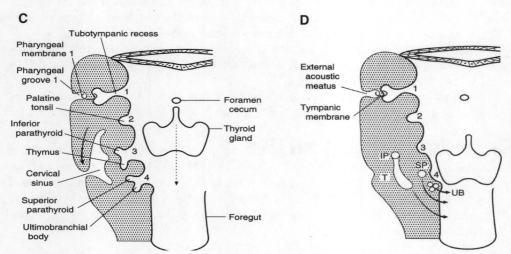

● **Figure 12.1 (A) Lateral view of an embryo in week 4 of development, showing the pharyngeal arches.** Note that pharyngeal arch 1 consists of a maxillary prominence and a mandibular prominence, which can cause some confusion in numbering of the arches. **(B) A schematic diagram indicating a convenient way to understand the numbering of the arches and pouches.** The X's indicate regression of pharyngeal arch 5 and pouch 5. **(C and D) Schematic diagrams of the fate of the pharyngeal pouches, grooves, and membranes. (C)** Solid arrow indicates the downward growth of pharyngeal arch 2, thereby forming a smooth contour at the neck region. Dotted arrow indicates downward migration of the thyroid gland. **(D)** Curved arrows indicate direction of migration of the inferior parathyroid (IP), thymus (T), superior parathyroid (SP), and ultimobranchial bodies (UB). Note that the parathyroid tissue derived from pharyngeal pouch 3 is carried farther caudally by the descent of the thymus than parathyroid tissue from pharyngeal pouch 4.

B. **The pharyngeal part (posterior third) of the tongue** forms from the **copula** and **hypobranchial eminence**, which develop in the floor of the pharynx associated with **pharyngeal arches 2, 3, and 4.** The hypobranchial eminence overgrows the copula, thereby eliminating any contribution of pharyngeal arch 2 in the formation of the definitive adult tongue. The line of fusion between the oral and pharyngeal parts of the tongue is indicated by the **terminal sulcus.** The pharyngeal part is characterized by the **lingual tonsil,** which forms along with the palatine tonsil and pharyngeal tonsil (adenoids) **Waldeyer's ring.** General sensation from the mucosa is carried primarily by the **glossopharyngeal nerve (CN IX).** Taste sensation is carried predominantly by the **glossopharyngeal nerve (CN IX).**

C. **Muscles of the tongue.** The intrinsic and extrinsic muscles (styloglossus, hyoglossus, genioglossus, and palatoglossus) are derived from myoblasts that migrate into the tongue region from **occipital somites.** Motor innervation is supplied by the **hypoglossal nerve (CN XII)** except for the palatoglossus muscle, which is innervated by CN X.

IV **Development of the Face** (Figure 12-2B). The face is formed by three swellings: the **frontonasal prominence, maxillary prominence** (pharyngeal arch 1), and **mandibular prominence** (pharyngeal arch 1). Bilateral ectodermal thickenings, called **nasal placodes,** develop on the ventrolateral aspects of the frontonasal prominence. The nasal placodes invaginate into the underlying mesoderm to form the **nasal pits,** thereby producing a ridge of tissue that forms the **medial** and **lateral nasal prominences.** A deep groove called the **nasolacrimal groove** forms between the maxillary prominence and the lateral nasal prominence, and eventually forming the **nasolacrimal duct** and **lacrimal sac.**

V **Development of the Palate** (Figure 12-2C)

A. **The intermaxillary segment** forms when the medial growth of the maxillary prominences causes the two medial nasal prominences to fuse together at the midline. The intermaxillary segment forms the **philtrum of the lip, four incisor teeth,** and **primary palate.**

B. **The secondary palate** forms from outgrowths of the maxillary prominences called the **palatine shelves.** Initially the palatine shelves project downward on either side of the tongue, but later they attain a horizontal position and fuse along the **palatine raphe** to form the **secondary palate.** The primary and secondary palates fuse at the **incisive foramen** to form the **definitive palate.** Bone develops in both the primary palate and anterior part of the secondary palate. Bone does not develop in the posterior part of the secondary palate, which eventually forms the **soft palate** and **uvula.** The **nasal septum** develops from the medionasal prominences and fuses with the definitive palate.

VI **Development of the Mouth.** The mouth is formed from a surface depression called the **stomodeum,** which is lined by ectoderm, and the **cephalic end of the foregut** which is lined by endoderm. The stomodeum and foregut meet at the **oropharyngeal membrane.** The epithelium of the **oral part of the tongue, hard palate, sides of the mouth, lips, parotid gland and ducts, Rathke's pouch,** and **enamel of the teeth** is derived from ectoderm. The epithelium of the **pharyngeal part of the tongue, floor of the mouth, palatoglossal fold, palatopharyngeal fold, soft palate, sublingual gland and ducts,** and **submandibular gland and ducts** is derived from endoderm.

VII **Clinical Correlations** (Figure 12-3)

A. **First arch syndrome** results from abnormal development of **pharyngeal arch 1** and produces various facial anomalies. It is caused by a lack of migration of neural crest cells into pharyngeal arch 1. Two well-described first arch syndromes are **Treacher Collins syndrome (mandibulofacial dysostosis)** and **Pierre Robin syndrome.**

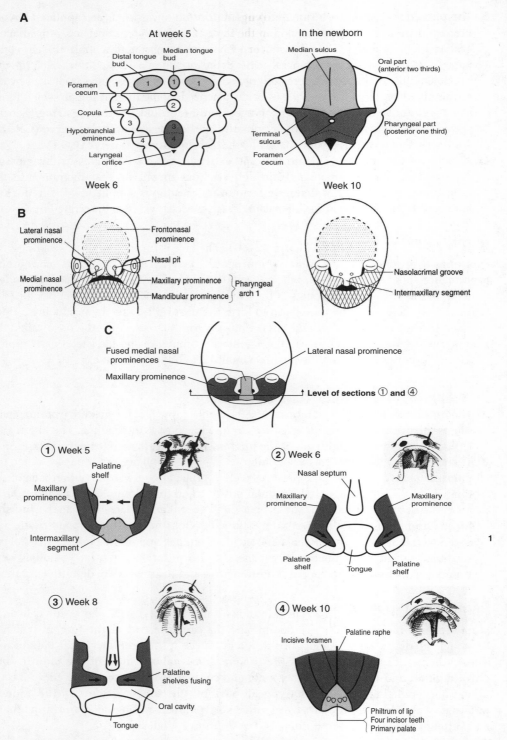

● **Figure 12.2 (A) Development of the tongue at week 5 and in the newborn. (B) Development of the face at weeks 6 and 10. (C) Development of the palate from weeks 5 through 10.** (1) Horizontal section as indicated shows the intermaxillary segment and maxillary prominence with palatine shelves growing toward the midline (arrows). (2 and 3) Coronal sections showing movements of the palatine shelves (single arrows) and fusion with the nasal septum (double arrows). (4) A horizontal section as indicated of the adult palate. Insets for 1–4 show the roof of the mouth. Arrows indicate open communication between the nasal cavities and mouth. Level of sections in 1 and 4 is noted in top drawing.

B. **Pharyngeal fistula** occurs when **pharyngeal pouch 2** and **pharyngeal groove 2** persist, thereby forming a patent opening from the internal tonsillar area to the external neck. It is generally found along the **anterior border of the sternocleidomastoid muscle.**

C. **Pharyngeal cyst** occurs when parts of the **pharyngeal grooves 2, 3, and 4,** which are normally obliterated, persist, thereby forming a cyst. It is generally found near the **angle of the mandible.**

D. **Ectopic thymus, parathyroid, or thyroid tissue** result from the abnormal migration of these glands from their embryonic position to their definitive adult location. Glandular tissue may be found anywhere along their migratory path.

E. **Thyroglossal duct cyst** occurs when parts of the thyroglossal duct persist and thus form a cyst. It is most commonly located in the midline near the hyoid bone but may also be located at the base of the tongue; it is then called a **lingual cyst.**

F. **Congenital hypothyroidism (cretinism)** occurs when a thyroid deficiency exists during the early fetal period due to either a severe lack of dietary iodine, thyroid agenesis, or mutations involving the biosynthesis of thyroid hormone. This condition causes impaired skeletal growth and mental retardation. It is characterized by coarse facial features; a low-set hairline; sparse eyebrows; wide-set eyes; periorbital puffiness; a flat, broad nose; an enlarged, protuberant tongue; a hoarse cry; umbilical hernia; dry, cold extremities; and dry, rough, mottled skin (myxedema). It is important to note that the majority of infants with congenital hypothyroidism have no physical stigmata. This has led to the screening of all newborns in the United States and in most other developed countries for levels of depressed thyroxin or elevated levels of thyroid-stimulating hormone.

G. **Cleft palate** has multifactorial causes, including participation of neural crest cells. It is classified as anterior or posterior. The anatomic landmark that separates anterior from posterior cleft palate defects is the incisive foramen.

   1. **Anterior cleft palate** occurs when the palatine shelves fail to fuse with the primary palate.
   2. **Posterior cleft palate** occurs when the palatine shelves fail to fuse with each other and with the nasal septum.
   3. **Anteroposterior cleft palate** occurs when there is a combination of both defects.

H. **Cleft lip** has multifactorial causes including the participation of neural crest cells. Cleft lip and cleft palate are distinct malformations based on their embryological formation, even though they often occur together. They may occur unilaterally or bilaterally. Unilateral cleft lip is the most common congenital malformation of the head and neck. It results from the following:

   1. The maxillary prominence fails to fuse with the medial nasal prominence.
   2. The underlying somitomeric mesoderm and neural crest fail to expand, resulting in a **persistent labial groove.**

I. **DiGeorge syndrome (DS)** occurs when **pharyngeal pouches 3 and 4** fail to differentiate into the thymus and parathyroid glands. DS is usually accompanied by facial anomalies resembling first arch syndrome (micrognathia, low-set ears) due to abnormal neural crest cell migration, cardiovascular anomalies due to abnormal neural crest cell migration during formation of the aorticopulmonary septum, immunodeficiency due to absence of the thymus gland, and hypocalcemia due to the absence of parathyroid glands.

J. **Ankyloglossia** (tongue-tie) occurs when the frenulum of the tongue extends to the tip of the tongue, thereby preventing protrusion.

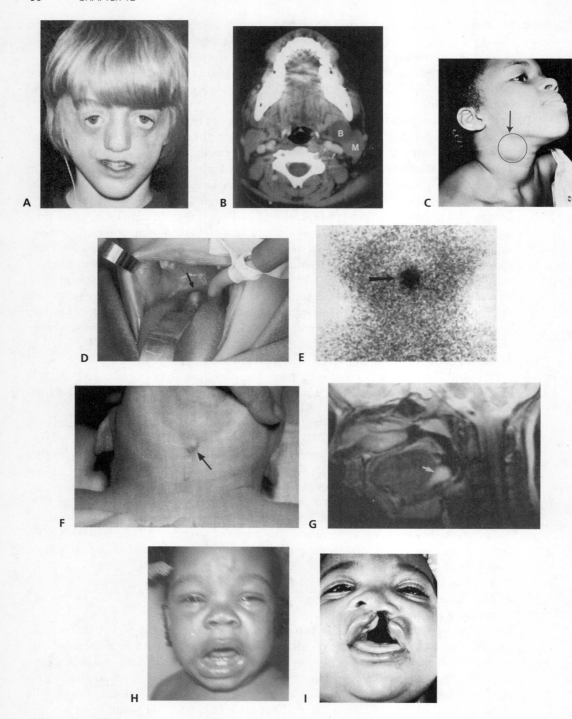

● **Figure 12.3 (A) Treacher Collins syndrome (mandibulofacial dysostosis).** Treacher Collins syndrome is characterized by underdevelopment of the zygomatic bones, mandibular hypoplasia, lower eyelid colobomas, downward-slanting palpebral fissures, and malformed external ears (note the hearing aid cord). This is an autosomal dominant genetic disorder involving a gene locus on chromosome 5q31.3-q33.3. **(B) Pharyngeal cyst/fistula.** A CT scan shows a low-density mass (B) just anteromedial to the sternocleidomastoid muscle (M) and anterolateral to the carotid artery and jugular vein (arrows). The pharyngeal cyst arises from a persistence of pharyngeal groove 2. This may also involve the persistence of pharyngeal pouch 2, thereby forming a patent opening of the fistula through the neck. The fistula may begin inside the throat near the tonsils, travel through the neck, and open to the outside near the anterior border of the sternocleidomastoid muscle. **(C) Pharyngeal cyst.** A fluid-filled cyst (circle) near the angle of the mandible (arrow). **(D, E) Ectopic thyroid tissue.** A sublingual

Case Study

While delivering a baby girl, you notice that she has abnormal facies as well as a cleft palate. What is the most likely diagnosis?

Differentials

- First arch syndrome, DiGeorge syndrome

Relevant Physical Exam Findings

- No detectable thymus upon palpation
- Cleft palate
- Muscular rigidity

Relevant Lab Findings

- Hypocalcemia
- X-ray indicates congenital heart disease
- Genetic testing shows a 22q deletion

Diagnosis

- DiGeorge syndrome. A first arch syndrome shows abnormal facies and cleft palate. However, DiGeorge syndrome presents with those conditions as well as hypocalcemia, 22q deletion, and tetany.

thyroid mass (arrow) is seen in this young euthyroid child. Nuclear scintigraphy localizes the position and the extent of the sublingual thyroid gland (arrow). There was no evidence of functioning thyroid tissue in the lower neck (i.e., normal anatomical position). **(F) Thyroglossal duct cyst.** A thyroglossal duct cyst (arrow) is one of the most frequent congenital anomalies in the neck and is found along the midline most frequently below the hyoid bone. **(G) Lingual cyst.** MRI shows a mass of thyroid tissue (arrow) at the base of the tongue. **(H) Congenital hypothyroidism (cretinism).** This condition causes impaired skeletal growth and mental retardation. This condition is characterized by coarse facial features; a low-set hairline; sparse eyebrows; wide-set eyes; periorbital puffiness; a flat, broad nose; an enlarged, protuberant tongue; a hoarse cry; umbilical hernia; dry, cold extremities; dry, rough, and mottled skin (myxedema). **(I) Unilateral cleft lip and cleft palate.**

Chapter 13

Nervous System

I Overview

A. The central nervous system (CNS) is formed in week 3 of development as the **neural plate.** The neural plate consisting of **neuroectoderm** becomes the **neural tube,** which gives rise to the brain and spinal cord.

B. The peripheral nervous system (PNS) is derived from three sources:
1. **Neural crest cells**
2. **Neural tube,** which gives rise to all preganglionic autonomic fibers and all fibers that innervate skeletal muscles.
3. **Mesoderm,** which gives rise to the dura mater and to connective tissue investments of peripheral nerve fibers (endoneurium, perineurium, and epineurium).

II Development of the Neural Tube (Figure 13-1).   **Neurulation** refers to the formation

and closure of the neural tube. The events of neurulation occur as follows:

A. The **notochord** induces the overlying ectoderm to differentiate into **neuroectoderm** and form the **neural plate.** The notochord forms the **nucleus pulposus** of the intervertebral disk in the adult.

B. The neural plate folds to give rise to the **neural tube,** which is open at both ends at the **anterior** and **posterior neuropores.** The anterior and posterior neuropores connect the lumen of the neural tube with the amniotic cavity.
1. The **anterior neuropore** closes during week 4 (day 25) and becomes the **lamina terminalis.** Failure of the anterior neuropore to close results in upper neural tube defects (NTDs; e.g., **anencephaly**).
2. The **posterior neuropore** closes during week 4 (day 27). Failure of the posterior neuropore to close results in lower NTDs (e.g., **spina bifida with myeloschisis**).

C. As the neural plate folds, some cells differentiate into **neural crest cells.**

D. The rostral part of the neural tube becomes the adult **brain.**

E. The caudal part of the neural tube becomes the adult **spinal cord.**

F. The lumen of the neural tube gives rise to the **ventricular system** of the brain and **central canal** of the spinal cord.

III Neural Crest Cells (Figure 13-1).   The neural crest cells differentiate from cells located

along the lateral border of the neural plate, a process is mediated by **BMP-4** (bone morphogenic protein) and **BMP-7.** The differentiation of neural crest cells is marked by the expression of *slug* (a zinc-finger transcription factor), which characterizes cells that break away from the neuroepithelium of the neural plate and migrate into the extracellular matrix as mesenchymal cells. Neural crest cells experience an extracellular environment rich in extracellular matrix molecules. Molecules that promote cell migration are **fibronectin, laminin,** and **type IV collagen.** Molecules that restrict cell migration are **chondroitin sulfate–rich proteoglycans.** Neural crest cells undergo a prolific migration throughout the

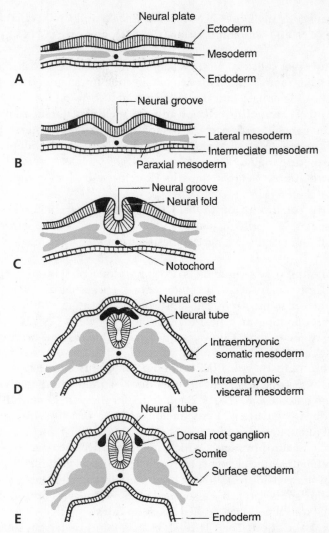

● **Figure 13.1 Schematic diagrams of transverse sections of embryos at various stages. (A)** Neural plate stage.
(B) Early neural groove stage. **(C)** Late neural groove stage. **(D)** Early neural tube and neural crest stage. **(E)** Neural tube and dorsal root ganglion stage.

embryo (both the cranial and trunk regions) and ultimately differentiate into a wide array of adult cells and structures.

A. Cranial neural crest cells. There is a remarkable relationship between the origin of cranial neural crest cells from the rhombencephalon (hindbrain) and their final migration into pharyngeal arches. The rhombencephalon is divided into eight segments called **rhombomeres (R1–R8).** Cranial neural crest cells from R1 and R2 migrate into pharyngeal arch 1 (which also receives neural crest cells from the midbrain area). Cranial neural crest cells from R4 migrate into pharyngeal arch 2. Cranial neural crest cells from R6 and R7 migrate into pharyngeal arch 3. This pattern seems to be controlled by the expression of the *Hoxb* **gene complex** and **OTX2.** Cranial neural crest cells differentiate into the following adult cells and structures: **pharyngeal arch skeletal and connective tissue components; bones of neurocranium; pia and arachnoid; parafollicular (C) cells of thyroid; aorticopulmonary septum; odontoblasts (dentin**

of teeth); sensory ganglia of CN V, CN VII, CN IX, and CN X; ciliary (CN III), ptery-gopalatine (CN VII), submandibular (CN VII), and otic (CN IX) parasympathetic ganglia.

B. **Trunk neural crest cells** extend from somite 6 to the most caudal somites and migrate in a dorsolateral, ventral, and ventrolateral direction throughout the embryo. Trunk neural crest cells differentiate into the following adult cells and structures: **melanocytes, Schwann cells, chromaffin cells of adrenal medulla, dorsal root ganglia, sympathetic chain ganglia, prevertebral sympathetic ganglia, enteric parasympathetic ganglia of the gut (Meissner and Auerbach; CN X), and abdominal/pelvic cavity parasympathetic ganglia.**

C. **Clinical correlations. Neurocristopathy** describes any disease related to maldevelopment of neural crest cells.

   1. **Medullary carcinoma of thyroid (MC).** MC is an endocrine neoplasm of the parafollicular (C) cells of neural crest origin that secrete calcitonin. The carcinoma cells are usually arranged in nests surrounded by bands of stroma containing amyloid.

   2. **Schwannoma.** A schwannoma is a benign tumor of Schwann cells of neural crest origin. These tumors are well-circumscribed, encapsulated masses that may or may not be attached to the nerve. The most common location within the cranial vault is at the cerebellopontine angle near the vestibular branch of CN VIII (often referred to as an **acoustic neuroma**). Clinical signs include tinnitus and hearing loss. CN V (the trigeminal nerve) is also commonly affected.

   3. **Neurofibromatosis type 1 (NF1; von Recklinghausen disease).** NF1 is a relatively common autosomal dominant disorder due to a mutation in the **NF1 gene,** which is located on chromosome 17q11.2 and codes for the protein **neurofibromin.** Neurofibromin down-regulates **p21 ras oncoprotein,** so that the NF1 gene belongs to the family of tumor-suppressor genes. The key features of NF include multiple neural tumors (called **neurofibromas**), **which** are widely dispersed over the body and reveal a proliferation of all the elements of a peripheral nerve, including neurites, fibroblasts, and Schwann cells of neural crest origin, numerous pigmented skin lesions (called **café-au-lait spots**) probably associated with melanocytes of neural crest origin, and pigmented iris hamartomas (called **Lisch nodules**).

   4. **CHARGE association.** The CHARGE association is understandable only if the wide distribution of neural crest cell derivatives is appreciated. The cause of CHARGE is unknown but seems to involve an insult during the second month of gestation probably involving the neural crest cells. The key features of CHARGE include **c**oloboma of the retina, lens, or choroid; **h**eart defects [e.g., tetralogy of Fallot, ventricular septal defect (VSD), patent ductus arteriosus (PDA)]; **a**tresia choanae; **r**etardation of growth; **g**enital abnormalities in male infants (e.g., cryptorchidism, microphallus); and **e**ar abnormalities or deafness.

   5. **Waardenburg syndrome (WS).** WS is an autosomal dominant disorder due to a mutation in either the **PAX3 gene,** which is located on chromosome 2q35 (for type I WS), or the **MITF gene,** which is located on chromosome 3p12.3-p14.1 (for type II WS). The key features of WS include lateral displacement of lacrimal puncta, a broad nasal root, heterochromia of the iris, congenital deafness, and piebaldism, including a white forelock and a triangular area of hypopigmentation.

   6. **Hirschsprung disease.**
   7. **Cleft palate and lip.**
   8. **DiGeorge syndrome.**
   9. **Pheochromocytoma.**
   10. **Neuroblastoma.**

Vesicular Development of the Neural Tube (Figure 13-2)

A. The three **primary brain vesicles** and two associated **flexures** develop during week 4.

 1. The **prosencephalon (forebrain)** is associated with the appearance of the **optic vesicles** and gives rise to the **telencephalon** and **diencephalon.**

 2. The **mesencephalon (midbrain)** remains as the **mesencephalon.**

 3. The **rhombencephalon (hindbrain)** gives rise to the **metencephalon** and **myelencephalon.**

 4. The **cephalic flexure (midbrain flexure)** is located between the prosencephalon and rhombencephalon.

 5. The **cervical flexure** is located between the rhombencephalon and the future spinal cord.

B. The five **secondary brain vesicles** become visible in week 6 of development and form various adult derivatives of the brain.

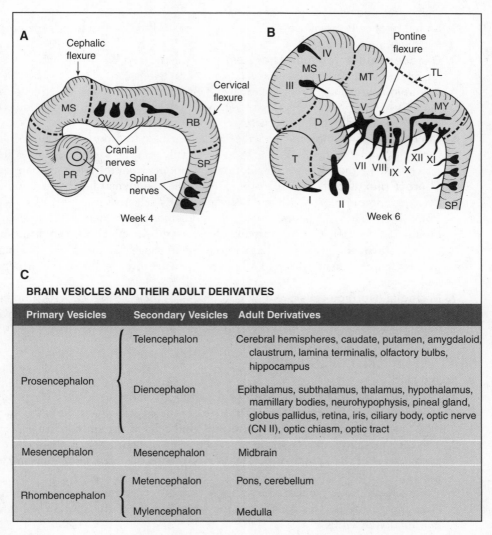

BRAIN VESICLES AND THEIR ADULT DERIVATIVES

Primary Vesicles	Secondary Vesicles	Adult Derivatives
Prosencephalon	Telencephalon	Cerebral hemispheres, caudate, putamen, amygdaloid, claustrum, lamina terminalis, olfactory bulbs, hippocampus
	Diencephalon	Epithalamus, subthalamus, thalamus, hypothalamus, mamillary bodies, neurohypophysis, pineal gland, globus pallidus, retina, iris, ciliary body, optic nerve (CN II), optic chiasm, optic tract
Mesencephalon	Mesencephalon	Midbrain
Rhombencephalon	Metencephalon	Pons, cerebellum
	Mylencephalon	Medulla

● **Figure 13.2 Schematic illustrations of the developing brain vesicles. (A)** Three-vesicle stage of the brain in a 4-week-old embryo. Divisions are indicated by dotted lines. PR = prosencephalon, MS = mesencephalon, RB = rhomben-cephalon, SP = spinal cord, OV = optic vesicle. **(B)** Five-vesicle stage of the brain in a 6-week-old embryo. Divisions are indicated by dotted lines. Cranial nerves (CN) are indicated by Roman numerals. CN VI is not shown because it exits the brainstem from the ventral surface. T = telencephalon, D = diencephalons, MS = mesencephalon, MT = metencephalon, MY = myelencephalon, TL = tela choroidea, SP = spinal cord. **(C)** Table indicating the brain vesicles and their adult derivatives.

Histogenesis of the Neural Tube. The cells of the neural tube are neuroectodermal (or neuroepithelial) cells that give rise to the following cell types:

A. Neuroblasts form all neurons found in the CNS.

B. Glioblasts (spongioblasts) are, for the most part, formed after cessation of neuroblast formation. Radial glial cells are an exception and develop before neurogenesis is complete. Glioblasts form the supporting cells of the CNS and include:

1. **Astroglia (astrocytes),** which have the following characteristics and functions: they project foot processes to capillaries that contribute to the blood-brain barrier, play a role in the metabolism of neurotransmitters (e.g., glutamate, GABA, serotonin), buffer the [K+] of the CNS extracellular space, form the external and internal glial-limiting membrane in the CNS, form glial scars in a damaged area of the CNS (i.e., astrogliosis), undergo hypertrophy and hyperplasia in reaction to CNS injury, contain the **glial fibrillary acidic protein (GFAP)** and **glutamine synthetase,** which are good markers for astrocytes.

2. **Radial glial cells** are of astrocytic lineage, are GFAP-positive, and provide guidance for migrating neuroblasts.

3. **Oligodendroglia (oligodendrocytes)** produce the **myelin** in the CNS. A single oligodendrocyte can myelinate several (up to 30) axons.

4. **Ependymocytes** line the central canal and ventricles of the brain. These cells are not joined by tight junctions, so that exchange between the cerebrospinal fluid (CSF) and CNS extracellular fluid occurs freely.

5. **Tanycytes** are modified ependymal cells that mediate transport between CSF in the ventricles and the neuropil. These cells usually project to hypothalamic nuclei, which regulate the release of gonadotropic hormones from the adenohypophysis.

6. **Choroid plexus cells** are a continuation of the ependymal layer that is reflected over the choroid plexus villi and **secrete CSF** by selective transport of molecules from blood. These cells are joined by tight junctions, which is the basis of the **blood-CSF barrier.** CSF is normally **clear.** A **yellow color (xanthochromia)** indicates previous bleeding (subarachnoid hemorrhage) or increased [protein]. A **pinkish color** is usually due to a bloody tap. **Turbidity** is due to the presence of leukocytes.

7. **Microglia (Hortega cells)** are the macrophages of the CNS, which arise from monocytes and invade the developing nervous system in week 3, along with the developing blood vessels.

Layers of the Early Neural Tube

A. Spinal cord

1. The **ventricular zone (neuroepithelial layer)** gives rise to a layer of ependymal cells, which line the central canal. The neuroepithelial cells migrate into the intermediate layer and give rise to all **neurons and glial cells of the spinal cord.**

2. The **intermediate zone (mantle layer)** consists of neurons and glial cells of the **gray matter of the spinal cord.** This zone contains the developing **alar** and **basal plates.**

3. The **marginal zone** contains nerve fibers (axons) of the neuroblasts of the mantle layer and glial cells. This zone forms the **white matter of the spinal cord** through myelination of axons.

B. Brain

1. The **ventricular zone (neuroepithelial layer)** gives rise to a layer of ependymal cells, which line the ventricles, and to all **neurons and glial cells of the brain.**

2. The **intermediate zone (mantle layer),** along with the ventricular layer, gives rise to the **cerebral cortex** and **basal ganglia.**

3. The **marginal zone** becomes the molecular layer of the cortex, which underlies the pia.

4. The **cortex** is the **gray matter** of the cerebral hemispheres.

VII **Development of the Spinal Cord.**   The spinal cord develops from the neural tube caudal to the fourth pair of somites.

A. The **alar (sensory) plate** is a **dorsolateral** thickening of the intermediate zone (mantle layer) of the neural tube and gives rise to **sensory neuroblasts of the dorsal horn** [general somatic afferent (GSA) and general visceral afferent (GVA) cell regions]. The alar plate receives axons from the dorsal root ganglia, which enter the spinal cord and become the **dorsal (sensory) roots.** The alar plate eventually becomes the **dorsal horn of the spinal cord.**

B. The **basal (motor) plate** is a **ventrolateral** thickening of the intermediate zone (mantle layer) of the neural tube and gives rise to **motor neuroblasts of the ventral and lateral horns** [general somatic efferent (GSE) and general visceral efferent (GVE) cell regions]. The basal plate projects axons from motor neuroblasts, which exit the spinal cord and become the **ventral (motor) roots.** The basal plate eventually becomes the **ventral horn of the spinal cord.**

C. The **sulcus limitans (SL)** is a **longitudinal groove** in the lateral wall of the neural tube that appears during week 4 of development and separates the alar and basal plates. The SL disappears in the adult spinal cord but is retained in the rhomboid fossa of the brainstem. The SL extends from the spinal cord to the rostral midbrain.

D. The **roof plate** is the nonneural roof of the central canal, which connects the two alar plates.

E. The **floor plate** is the nonneural floor of the central canal, which connects the two basal plates. The floor plate contains the ventral white commissure.

F. The **caudal eminence** arises from the primitive streak and blends with the neural tube. The caudal eminence gives rise to **sacral and coccygeal segments of the spinal cord.**

G. **Myelination** of the spinal cord begins during month 4 in the ventral (motor) roots. **Oligodendrocytes** accomplish myelination in the **CNS** and **Schwann cells** accomplish myelination in the **PNS.** Myelination of the corticospinal tracts is not completed until the child reaches 2 years of age (i.e., when the corticospinal tracts become myelinated and functional). Myelination of the **association neocortex** extends to 30 years of age.

H. **Positional changes of the spinal cord (Figure 13-3A). At week 8** of development, the spinal cord extends the length of the vertebral canal. **At birth,** the **conus medullaris** extends to the level of the third lumbar vertebra (**L3**). **In adults,** the conus medullaris terminates at the **L1–L2 interspace.** Disparate growth (between the vertebral column and the spinal cord) results in the formation of the **cauda equina,** consisting of dorsal and ventral roots, which descends below the level of the conus medullaris. Disparate growth results in the nonneural **filum terminale,** which anchors the spinal cord to the coccyx.

VIII **Development of the Hypophysis** (**pituitary gland; Figure 13-3B**).   The hypophysis is attached to the hypothalamus by the pituitary stalk and consists of two lobes.

A. The **anterior lobe (adenohypophysis), pars tuberalis,** and **pars intermedia** develop from **Rathke's pouch,** which is an ectodermal diverticulum of the primitive mouth cavity (stomodeum). Remnants of Rathke's pouch may give rise to a **craniopharyngioma.**

B. The **posterior lobe (neurohypophysis)** develops from a ventral evagination of the hypothalamus. The posterior lobe includes the **median eminence, infundibular stem,** and **pars nervosa.**

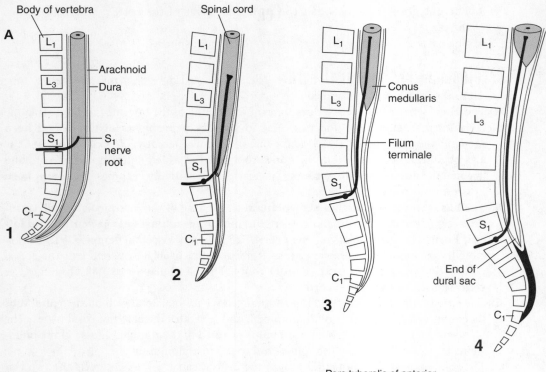

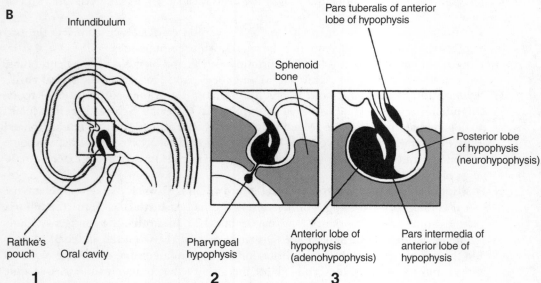

● **Figure 13.3 (A) Positional changes in the spinal cord.** The end of the spinal cord (conus medullaris) is shown in relation to the vertebral column and meninges. (1) Week 8. (2) Week 24. (3) Newborn. (4) Adult. As the vertebral column grows, nerve roots (especially those of the lumbar and sacral segments) are elongated to form the cauda equina. The S1 nerve root is shown as an example. **(B) Development of the hypophysis.** (1) A midsagittal section through a week-6 embryo showing Rathke's pouch as a dorsal outpocketing of the oral cavity and the infundibulum as a thickening in the floor of the hypothalamus. (2,3) Development at weeks 11 and 16, respectively. The anterior lobe, pars tuberalis, and pars intermedia are derived from Rathke's pouch.

IX # Congenital Malformations of the Central Nervous System

A. Variations of spina bifida (Figure 13-4). Spina bifida occurs when the **bony vertebral arches** fail to form properly, thereby creating a vertebral defect usually in the **lumbosacral region.** It is due primarily to the failure of expectant mothers to take enough folic acid during pregnancy.

1. **Spina bifida occulta** is evidenced by a tuft of hair in the lumbosacral region. It is the least severe variation and occurs in 10% of the population.
2. **Spina bifida with meningocele** occurs when the meninges protrude through a vertebral defect and form a sac filled with CSF. The spinal cord remains in its normal position.
3. **Spina bifida with meningomyelocele** occurs when the meninges and spinal cord protrude through a vertebral defect and form a sac filled with CSF.
4. **Spina bifida with rachischisis** occurs when the posterior neuropore of the neural tube fails to close during week 4 of development. This condition is the most severe type of spina bifida, causing paralysis from the level of the defect caudally. This variation presents clinically as an **open neural tube** that lies on the surface of the back. It also falls into a classification called **neural tube defects (NTDs). Lower NTDs** (i.e., spina bifida with rachischisis) result from a failure of the **posterior neuropore** to close during week 4 of development and usually occur in the lumbosacral region. **Upper NTDs** (e.g., anencephaly) result from a failure of the **anterior neuropore** to close during week 4 of development. NTDs can be diagnosed prenatally by detecting elevated levels of **α-fetoprotein** in the amniotic fluid. About 75% of all NTDs would be prevented if all women capable of becoming pregnant consumed **folic acid** (dose: 0.4 mg/day).

B. Variations of cranium bifida (Figure 13-5). Cranium bifida occurs when the **bony skull** fails to form properly, thereby creating a skull defect usually in the **occipital region.** It is due primarily to the failure of expectant mothers to take enough folic acid during pregnancy.

1. **Cranium bifida with meningocele** occurs when the meninges protrude through the skull defect and form a sac filled with CSF.
2. **Cranium bifida with meningoencephalocele** occurs when the meninges and brain protrude through the skull defect and form a sac filled with CSF. This defect usually comes to medical attention within the infant's first few days or weeks of life. The outcome is poor (i.e., 75% of such infants die or are severely retarded).
3. **Cranium bifida with meningohydroencephalocele** occurs when the meninges, brain, and a portion of the ventricle protrude through the skull defect.

C. Anencephaly (meroanencephaly). Anencephaly is a type of **upper NTD** that occurs when the **anterior neuropore** fails to close during week 4 (day 25) of development. This results in failure of the brain to develop (although a rudimentary brain is present), failure of the lamina terminalis to form, and failure of the bony cranial vault to form. Anencephaly is incompatible with extrauterine life. If not stillborn, infants with anencephaly survive from only a few hours to a few weeks. Anencephaly is a common serious birth defect seen in stillborn fetuses. Anencephaly is easily diagnosed by ultrasound; when it is found, a therapeutic abortion is usually performed at the mother's request.

D. Arnold-Chiari malformation occurs when the caudal vermis and tonsils of the cerebellum and the medulla oblongata herniate through the foramen magnum. Clinical signs are caused by compression of the medulla oblongata and stretching of CN IX, CN X, and CN XII; they include spastic dysphonia, difficulty in swallowing, laryngeal stridor (a vibrating sound heard during respiration as a result of obstructed airways), diminished gag reflex, apnea, and vocal cord paralysis. This malformation is commonly associated with a **lumbar meningomyelocele, platybasia** (bone malformation of base of skull) along with malformation of the occipitovertebral joint, and **obstructive hydrocephalus** (due to obliteration of the foramen of Magendie and foramina of Luschka of the fourth ventricle; however, about 50% of cases demonstrate **aqueductal stenosis**).

E. **Hydrocephalus (Figure 13-6)** is a dilation of the ventricles due to an excess of CSF, which may result from either a blockage of the CSF circulation or, rarely, an overproduction of CSF (e.g., due to a choroid plexus papilloma). There are two general categories of hydrocephalus:

   1. **Communicating (or nonobstructive) hydrocephalus.** In this type of hydrocephalus, there is free communication between the ventricles and the subarachnoid space. The blockage of CSF in this type of hydrocephalus is usually in the subarachnoid space or arachnoid granulations, which results in the enlargement of all the ventricular cavities as well as the subarachnoid space.

   2. **Noncommunicating (or obstructive) hydrocephalus.** In this type of hydrocephalus, there is a lack of communication between the ventricles and the subarachnoid space. The blockage of CSF in this type of hydrocephalus is in the foramen of Monro, cerebral aqueduct, or foramen of Magendie/foramina of Luschka; this results in the enlargement of only those ventricular cavities proximal to the blockage. There are two types of **congenital hydrocephalus,** both of which produce a noncommunicating (obstructive) hydrocephalus:

      a. **Congenital aqueductal stenosis** is the most common cause of congenital hydrocephalus. This type may be transmitted by an X-linked trait, or it may be caused by cytomegalovirus or toxoplasmosis.

      b. **Dandy-Walker syndrome** appears to be associated with **atresia of the foramen of Magendie and foramina of Luschka** (although this remains controversial). It is usually associated with dilation of the fourth ventricle, posterior fossa cyst, agenesis of the cerebellar vermis, small cerebellar hemispheres, occipital meningocele, and frequently agenesis of the splenium of the corpus callosum.

F. **Porencephaly (encephaloclastic porencephaly; Figure 13-7A)** is the presence of one or more fluid-filled cystic cavities within the brain that may communicate with the ventricles but do not extend to the cerebral cortical surface. The cysts are lined by ependyma and have smooth or irregular walls. These cysts form as a result of brain destruction early in gestation, before the brain is capable of a glial response to form a scar.

G. **Hydranencephaly (Figure 13-7B,C)** is the presence of a huge, fluid-filled cystic cavity that completely replaces the cerebral hemispheres. The cyst is lined by glial and meningeal elements. This cystic cavity forms as a result of occlusion of the **internal carotid arteries** in utero, causing widespread destruction of the cerebral cortex (the brainstem and cerebellum are usually spared, since the vertebrobasilar circulation is not affected). Other causes include toxoplasmosis, rubella, cytomegalovirus, and herpesvirus.

H. **Schizencephaly (Figure 13-7D)** is the presence of a cerebral cortical cleft of brain tissue that extends from the ventricles to the cerebral cortical surface. The cleft is lined by cortical brain tissue and filled with fluid (i.e., it is a fluid-filled cleft). The cleft forms as a result of abnormal neuronal migration during embryological formation of the brain.

I. **Holoprosencephaly (arrhinencephaly; Figure 13-7E,F)** occurs when the prosencephalon fails to cleave down the midline, such that the telencephalon contains a single ventricle. It is characterized by the absence of olfactory bulbs and tracts (arrhinencephaly) and midline facial defects, including cyclops and the presence of a proboscis. It is often seen in trisomy 13 (Patau syndrome), trisomy 18 (Edward syndrome), short arm deletion of chromosome 18, Meckel syndrome, and in children of diabetic mothers. Because the fetal face develops at the same time as the brain, facial anomalies (e.g., cyclopia, cleft lip, cleft palate) are commonly seen with holoprosencephaly. Holoprosencephaly is the most severe manifestation of **fetal alcohol syndrome,** resulting from alcohol abuse during pregnancy (especially in the first 4 weeks of pregnancy). There are three types of holoprosencephaly, as indicated below:

1. **Alobar proencephaly** (most severe form) occurs when there is complete absence of cleavage of the prosencephalon. These infants are stillborn or die shortly after birth and have cyclopia, a single rudimentary proboscis, cleft lip, cleft palate, hypotelorism, and micrognathia. Sonographic findings include a single, horseshoe-shaped ventricle (monoventricle), fused thalami, and a pancake-like mantle of undifferentiated cerebral cortical tissue.

2. **Semilobar proencephaly** (intermediate form) occurs when there is absence of cleavage of the prosencephalon anteriorly, but partial cleavage of the prosencephalon posteriorly.

3. **Lobar proencephaly** (least severe form) occurs when there is absence of cleavage of the prosencephalon anteriorly but cleavage of the prosencephalon posteriorly.

J. Tethered spinal cord (filum terminale syndrome; Figure 13-7G) occurs when a thick, short filum terminale forms. The result is weakness and sensory deficits in the lower extremity and a neurogenic bladder. Tethered spinal cord is frequently associated with lipomatous tumors or meningomyeloceles. Deficits usually improve after transection.

K. A chordoma is a tumor that arises from remnants of the notochord.

Ⓧ **Selected Photographs, Sonograms, and Radiographs of Various Congenital Malformations**

A. Variations of spina bifida (Figure 13-4)
B. Variations of cranium bifida, anencephaly, and Arnold-Chiari malformation (Figure 13-5)
C. Communicating hydrocephalus, congenital aqueductal stenosis, and Dandy-Walker syndrome (Figure 13-6)
D. Porencephaly, hydranencephaly, schizencephaly, holoprosencephaly, and tethered spinal cord (Figure 13-7)

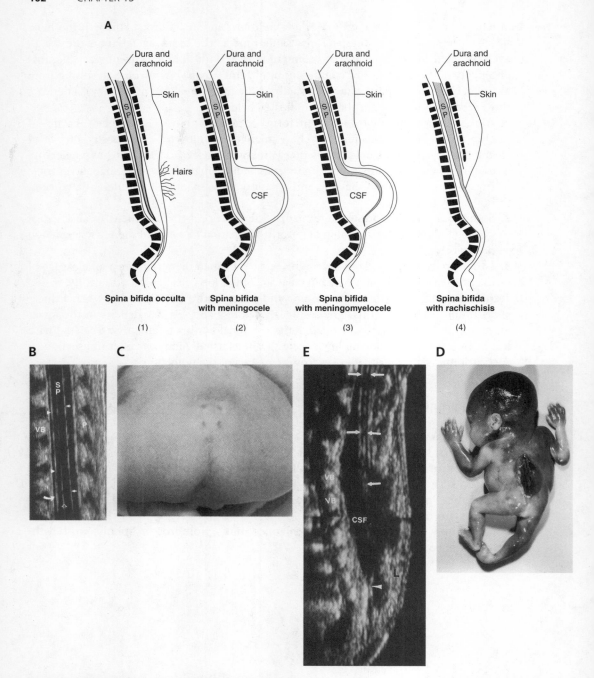

● **Figure 13.4 (A) Schematic drawings illustrating the various types of spina bifida.** (1) Spina bifida occulta. (2) Spina bifida with meningocele. (3) Spina bifida with meningomyelocele. (4) Spina bifida with rachischisis. **(B) Sonogram of a normal spinal cord in lower thoracic and upper lumbar region.** Note the vertebral bodies (VB), spinous processes (P), and spinal cord (SP) with its anterior median fissure (open arrow), posterior surface of the spinal cord (arrows), anterior surface of the spinal cord (arrowheads), and subarachnoid space containing cerebrospinal fluid (curved arrow). **(C) Spina bifida occulta.** Note the multiple dimples present on the back of the infant in the lumbosacral region, which may or may not be accompanied by a tuft of hair. In spina bifida occulta, the bony vertebral bodies are present along the entire length of the vertebral column. However, the bony spinous processes terminate at a much higher level, since the vertebral arches fail to form properly. This creates a bony vertebral defect. The spinal cord is intact. **(D) Spina bifida with meningomyelocele.** Note the spinal cord (arrows), cerebrospinal fluid (CSF)–filled sac, small subcutaneous lipoma (L), and filum terminale (arrowhead). **(E) Spina bifida with rachischisis.** Photograph of a newborn infant shows the open neural tube on the child's back.

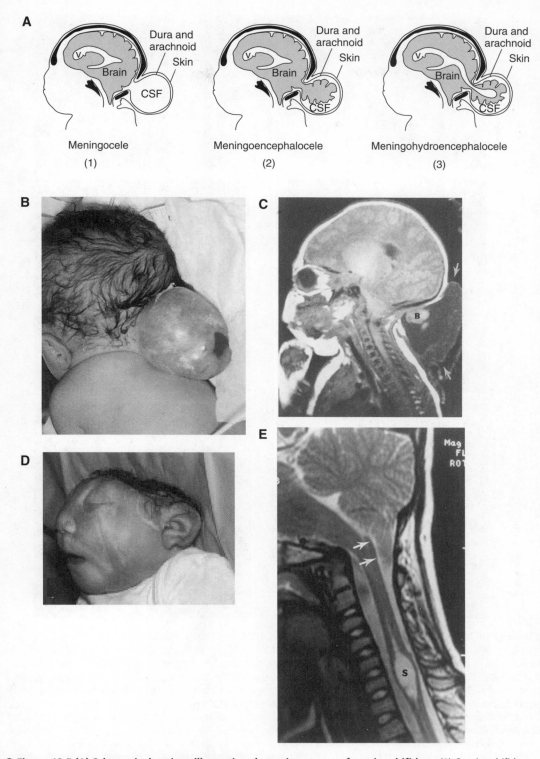

● **Figure 13.5 (A) Schematic drawings illustrating the various types of cranium bifidum.** (1) Cranium bifidum with meningocele. (2) Cranium bifidum with meningoencephalocele. (3) Cranium bifidum with meningohydroencephalocele. **(B) Photograph of a fetus with an occipital encephalocele. (C) MRI of a meningoencephalocele.** The MRI demonstrates a large encephalocele (arrows) extending through an occipital bone defect containing brain tissue (B). **(D) Photograph of a newborn infant with anencephaly. (E) MRI of an Arnold-Chiari malformation.** Note the herniation of the brainstem and cerebellum (arrows) through the foramen magnum. Note the presence of a syrinx (S) in the cervical spinal cord.

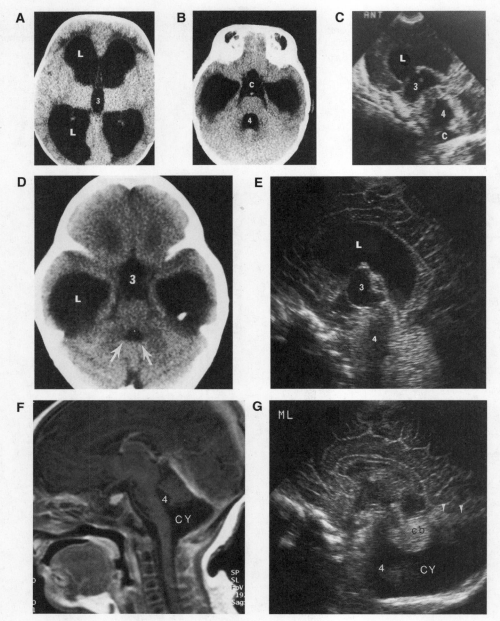

● **Figure 13.6 (A,B,C) Communicating hydrocephalus. (A)** CT scan shows dilated lateral ventricles (L) and a dilated third ventricle (3). **(B)** CT scan (lower level) shows a dilated fourth ventricle (4) and the cisterna magna (C).
(C) Sonogram shows the dilated lateral ventricle (L) communicating through a dilated foramen of Monro with a dilated
third ventricle (3) and dilated fourth ventricle (4). The cisterna magna (C) is also shown. **(D,E) Congenital aqueductal
stenosis. (D)** CT scan shows dilated lateral ventricles (L), dilated third ventricle (3), but normal-size fourth ventricle
(arrows). Therefore, obstruction at the cerebral aqueduct is presumed. **(E)** Sonogram shows dilated lateral ventricles (L),
dilated third ventricle (3), but normal-size fourth ventricle (4). Therefore, obstruction at the cerebral aqueduct is presumed.
(F,G) Dandy-Walker syndrome. (F) MRI shows a dilated fourth ventricle (4) communicating with a posterior fossa cyst
(CY) along with small cerebellar hemispheres. **(G)** Sonogram shows a massively dilated fourth ventricle (4) communicating with a large retrocerebellar fluid-filled cyst (CY) along with an elevated tentorium (arrowheads). A rudimentary cerebellar hemisphere (cb) can be observed.

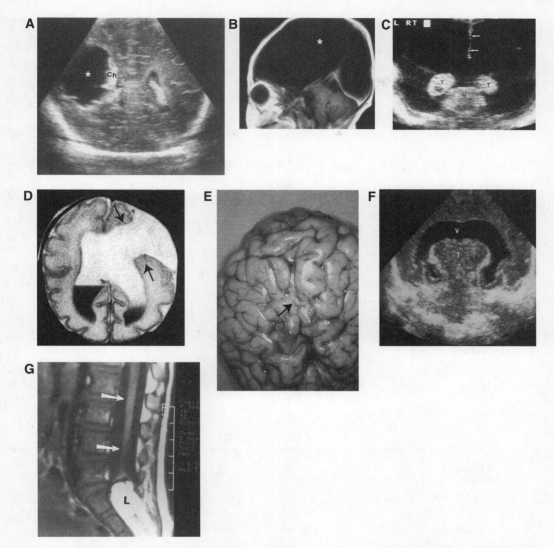

● **Figure 13.7 (A) Porencephaly.** Sonogram shows a fluid-filled cystic cavity (*) communicating with the right lateral ventricle. Ch = choroid plexus. **(B,C) Hydranencephaly. (B)** MRI shows a huge fluid-filled cystic cavity within the supratentorial compartment (*) which replaces the cerebral hemispheres. Note that the brainstem and cerebellum re-main intact. **(C)** Coronal sonogram shows a huge fluid-filled cystic cavity (*). Note that the thalami (T), cerebellar vermis (V), and falx cerebri (arrows) are normal. Compare this to holoprosencephaly. **(D) Schizencephaly.** MRI shows a cleft of brain tissue in the left cerebral hemisphere (arrows). This cleft is filled with fluid and communicates with the lat-eral ventricles. **(E,F) Holoprosencephaly.** (E) Superior photographic view of the brain shows failure of the prosen-cephalon to cleave down the midline and the absence of an anterior interhemispheric fissure. Note the single ventricle (V) surrounded by a mantle of cerebral cortical tissue, fused thalami (T), and absence of the falx cerebri. Compare this to hydranencephaly. **(F)** Sonogram shows a single horseshoe-shaped ventricle (V) and fused thalami (T). **(G) Tethered spinal cord.** MRI shows a low-positioned spinal cord (arrows) attached to an intraspinal lipoma (L).

Case Study 1

After delivery of a baby boy, you notice that the infant has microcephaly, polydactyly, and hypotelorism. The mother of the infant is 43 years old.

Differentials

- Down syndrome, Edwards syndrome, Patau syndrome

Relevant Physical Exam Findings

- Small head (microcephaly)
- Cleft lip and palate
- Polydactyly
- Close-set eyes (hypotelorism)
- Signs of congenital heart disease (ventricular septal defect, atrial septal defect)

Relevant Lab Findings

- Head CT shows holoprosencephaly
- Chromosome studies reveal trisomy 13

Diagnosis

- Patau syndrome

Case Study 2

After the delivery of a healthy baby girl, the physician notices a tuft of hair on the child's lower back. When he asks the mother about her prenatal health care, and she says that did not take a folic acid supplement until her second month because she didn't know she was pregnant until then.

Differentials

- Spina bifida occulta, spina bifida with meningocele, spina bifida with meningomyelocele

Relevant Physical Exam Findings

- Tuft of hair on lower back
- No noticeable sac formation

Relevant Lab Findings

- X-ray confirms that there is a defect in the vertebral arches; however, the exam is negative for a sac filled with fluid or spinal cord.

Diagnosis

- Spina bifida occulta is evidenced by the tuft of hair in the sacrolumbar region. Spina bifida of any type results from a lack of folic acid during the early period of pregnancy (i.e., around day 28 of pregnancy).

Chapter 14

Ear

I   **Overview.**   The ear is the organ of **balance** and **hearing**. It consists of an **internal**, a **middle**, and an **external ear.**

II   **The Internal Ear** (**Figure 14-1**) develops in week 4 from a thickening of the surface **ectoderm** called the **otic placode.** The otic placode invaginates into the connective tissue (mesenchyme) adjacent to the rhombencephalon and becomes the **otic vesicle.** The otic vesicle divides into **utricular** and **saccular portions.**

    A. The **utricular portion** of the otic vesicle gives rise to the:

        1. Utricle, which contains the sensory hair cells and otoliths of the macula utriculi. The utricle responds to **linear acceleration** and the **force of gravity.**

        2. Semicircular ducts, which contain the sensory hair cells of the cristae ampullares. They respond to **angular acceleration.**

        3. Vestibular ganglion of CN VIII, which lies at the base of the internal auditory meatus.

        4. Endolymphatic duct, a membranous duct that connects the saccule to the utricle, which terminates in the **endolymphatic sac,** a blind sac beneath the dura. The endolymphatic sac absorbs endolymph.

    B. The **saccular portion** of the otic vesicle gives rise to the:

        1. Saccule, which contains the sensory hair cells and otoliths of the macula sacculi. The saccule responds to **linear acceleration** and the **force of gravity.**

        2. Cochlear duct (organ of Corti), which is involved in hearing. This duct has pitch (tonopic) localization, whereby high-frequency sound waves (~20,000 Hz) are detected at the base and low frequency sound waves (~20 Hz) are detected at the apex.

        3. Spiral ganglion of CN VIII, which lies in the modiolus of the bony labyrinth.

III   **The Membranous and Bony Labyrinth.**   The membranous labyrinth consists of all the structures derived from the otic vesicle (Table 14-1). The membranous labyrinth is initially surrounded by neural crest cells, which form a connective tissue (mesenchyme) covering. This connective tissue becomes cartilaginous and then ossifies to become the **bony labyrinth** of the temporal bone. The connective tissue closest to the membranous labyrinth degenerates, thus forming the **perilymphatic space,** which contains **perilymph.** This sets up the interesting anatomical relationship whereby the membranous labyrinth is suspended (or floats) within the bony labyrinth by perilymph. Perilymph, which is similar in composition to **CSF,** communicates with the subarachnoid space via the **perilymphatic duct.**

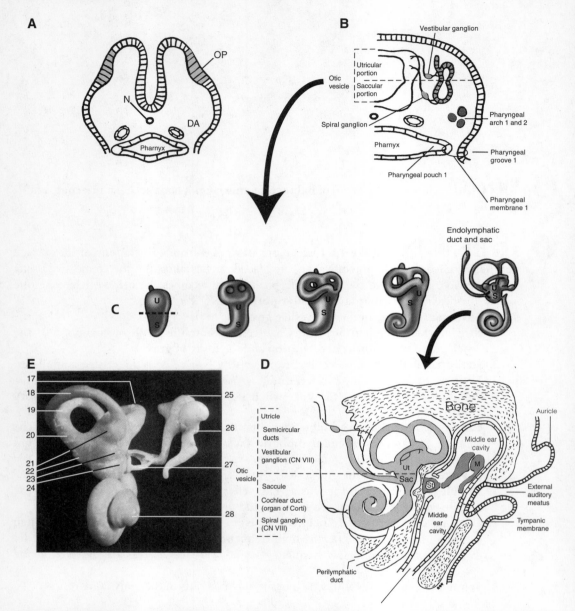

● **Figure 14.1 Schematic transverse sections showing the formation of the otic placode and otic vesicle from the surface ectoderm. (A)** The otic placode is distinguished by a thickening of the surface ectoderm. DA = dorsal aorta, N = notochord, OP = otic placode. **(B)** The otic placode invaginates into the underlying connective tissue (mesenchyme) and becomes the otic vesicle. **(C)** The otic vesicle undergoes extensive changes to form the adult membranous labyrinth. U = utricle, S = saccule. **(D)** The adult ear. M = malleus, St = stapes. **(E)** The adult auditory ossicles in connection with the bony labyrinth (or internal ear). 17 = lateral semicircular canal, 18 = anterior semicircular canal, 19 = posterior semicircular canal, 20 = common crus, 21 = ampulla, 22 = beginning of the endolymphatic duct, 23 = utricle, 24 = saccule, 25 = incus, 26 = malleus, 27 = stapes, 28 = cochlea.

IV Middle Ear (Figure 14-1)
A. **Ossicles of the middle ear**
  1. The malleus develops from cartilage of **pharyngeal arch 1** (Meckel's cartilage) and is attached to the tympanic membrane. The malleus is moved by the **tensor tympani muscle,** which is innervated by CN V_3.
  2. The **incus** develops from the cartilage of **pharyngeal arch 1** (Meckel's cartilage). The incus articulates with the malleus and stapes.
  3. The **stapes** develops from the cartilage of **pharyngeal arch 2** (Reichert's cartilage). The stapes is moved by the **stapedius** muscle, which is innervated by CN VII. It is attached to the oval window of the vestibule.
B. The **auditory tube and middle ear cavity** both develop from **pharyngeal pouch 1.**
C. The **tympanic membrane** develops from **pharyngeal membrane 1.** This membrane separates the middle ear from the external auditory meatus of the external ear. It is innervated by CN V_3 and CN IX.

V External Ear (Figure 14-1)
A. The **external auditory meatus** develops from **pharyngeal groove 1.** The meatus becomes filled with ectodermal cells, forming a temporary **meatal plug** that disappears before birth. The meatus is innervated by **CN V_3** and **CN IX.**
B. The **auricle (or pinna)** develops from **six auricular hillocks** that surround pharyngeal groove 1. The auricle is innervated by **CN V_3, CN VII, CN IX, and CN X,** and **cervical nerves C_2 and C_3.**

VI Congenital Malformations of the Ear (Figure 14-2)
A. **Minor auricular malformations** are commonly found and raise only cosmetic issues. However, auricular malformations are seen in **Down syndrome (trisomy 21), Patau syndrome (trisomy 13),** and **Edwards syndrome (trisomy 18).**
B. **Low-set, slanted auricles** are auricles that are located below a line extended from the corner of the eye to the occiput. This condition may indicate chromosomal abnormalities, as indicated above.
C. The **preauricular sinus** is a narrow tube or shallow pit that has a pinpoint external opening; it is most often asymptomatic and of minor cosmetic importance, although infections may occur. The embryological basis is uncertain but probably involves pharyngeal groove 1.
D. **Auricular appendages** are skin tags commonly found anterior to the auricle (i.e., the pretragal area), which raise only cosmetic issues. The embryological basis is the formation of accessory auricle hillocks.
E. **Atresia of the external auditory meatus.** A **complete atresia** consists of a bony plate in the location of the tympanic membrane. A **partial atresia** consists of a soft tissue plug in the location of the tympanic membrane. This results in conduction deafness and is usually associated with the first arch syndrome. The embryological basis is failure of the meatal plug to canalize.
F. **Congenital cholesteatoma** (epidermoid cyst) is a benign tumor found in the middle ear cavity; it results conduction deafness. The embryological basis is the proliferation of endodermal cells lining the middle ear cavity.
G. **Microtia** is a severely disorganized auricle associated with other malformations and resulting in deafness. The embryological basis is impaired proliferation or fusion of the auricular hillocks.
H. **Congenital deafness.** The organ of Corti may be damaged by exposure to **rubella virus,** especially during weeks 7 and 8 of development.

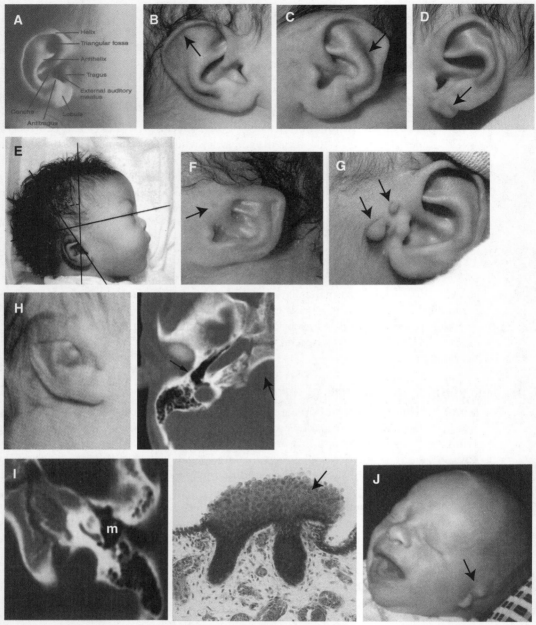

● **Figure 14.2 Congential malformations of the ear. (A)** Nomenclature of the adult auricle. **(B)** A minor auricular variation showing minimal folding of the helix (arrow), posterior rotation, and mildly low-set auricles. **(C)** A minor auricular variation showing a partially folded helix with a prominent antihelix (arrow). **(D)** A minor auricular variation showing a cleft lobule (arrow). **(E)** A severely low-set and posteriorly rotated auricle in an infant with Stickler syndrome. **(F)** A preauricular sinus is shown in the pretragal area. **(G)** Auricular appendages (i.e., skin tags) are shown in the pre-tragal area (arrows). **(H)** Atresia of the external auditory meatus. Photograph shows the absence of the external auditory meatus in this infant. CT scan shows microtia, absence of aerated external auditory meatus, and a bony plate (arrow) near the tympanic membrane. **(I)** Congenital cholesteatoma. CT scan shows a visible mass (m) behind the tympanic membrane (arrow). LM shows a large epidermoid formation (arrow). **(J)** Microtia shows a severely dis-organized auricle (arrow).

TABLE 14-1	EMBRYONIC EAR STRUCTURES AND THEIR ADULT DERIVATIVES
Embryonic Structure	**Adult Structure**
	Internal ear
Otic vesicle	
Utricular portion	Utricle, semicircular ducts, vestibular ganglion of CN VIII, endolymphatic duct and sac
Saccular portion	Saccule, cochlear duct (organ of Corti), spiral ganglion of CN VIII
	Middle ear
Pharyngeal arch 1	Malleus, incus, tensor tympani muscle
Pharyngeal arch 2	Stapes, stapedius muscle
Pharyngeal pouch 1	Auditory tube, middle ear cavity
Pharyngeal membrane 1	Tympanic membrane
	External ear
Pharyngeal groove 1	External auditory meatus
Auricular hillocks	Auricle

Case Study

A mother brings her 1-week-old son in to the clinic; she says that her son cannot seem to hear when she calls. She also reports that she was ill toward the beginning of her pregnancy and "broke out in a rash," but that this probably "was due to a new lotion she was using." What is the most likely diagnosis?

Differentials

• Congenital hearing defect

Relevant Physical Exam Findings

• Microcephaly
• Deafness
• Hepatosplenomegaly

Relevant Lab Findings

• Low platelet count
• CSF was positive for rubella

Diagnosis

• Rubella

Chapter **15**

Eye

❶ Development of the Optic Vesicle **(Figure 15-1; Table 15-1)** begins on day 22 with the formation of the **optic sulcus,** which evaginates from the wall of the diencephalon as the **optic vesicle,** consisting of **neuroectoderm.** The optic vesicle invaginates and forms a double-layered **optic cup** and **optic stalk. PAX6** is the master homeotic gene in eye development. PAX6 is expressed predominately in the optic cup and lens placode. **PAX2** is expressed predominately in the optic stalk.

A. The optic cup and its derivatives. The double-layered optic cup consists of an **outer pigment layer** and **inner neural layer.**

   1. Retina. The outer pigment layer of the optic cup gives rise to the **pigment layer of the retina.** The **intraretinal space** separates the outer pigment layer from the inner neural layer. Although the intraretinal space is obliterated in the adult, it remains a weakened area prone to **retinal detachment.** The inner neural layer of the otic cup gives rise to the **neural layer of the retina** (the rods and cones, bipolar cells, ganglion cells, etc.).

   2. Iris (Figure 15-2). The epithelium of the iris develops from the anterior portions of both the outer pigment layer and inner neural layer of the optic cup, which explains its histological appearance of two layers of columnar epithelium. The stroma develops from mesoderm continuous with the choroid. The iris contains the **dilator pupillae** and **sphincter pupillae muscles,** which are formed from the epithelium of the outer pigment layer by a transformation of these epithelial cells into contractile cells.

   3. The ciliary body (Figure 15-2). The epithelium of the ciliary body develops from the anterior portions of both the outer pigment layer and inner neural layer of the optic cup, which explains its histological appearance of two layers of columnar epithelium. The stroma develops from mesoderm continuous with the choroid. The ciliary body contains the **ciliary muscle,** which is formed from mesoderm within the choroid. The **ciliary processes** are components of the ciliary body.

      a. The ciliary processes produce **aqueous humor,** which circulates through the posterior and anterior chambers and drains into the venous circulation via the **trabecular meshwork** and the **canal of Schlemm.**

      b. The ciliary processes give rise to the **suspensory fibers** of the lens (ciliary zonule), which are attached to the lens and suspend it.

B. The optic stalk and its derivatives. The optic stalk contains the **choroid fissure,** in which the **hyaloid artery and vein** are found. The hyaloid artery and vein later become the **central artery and vein of the retina.** The optic stalk contains axons from the ganglion cell layer of the retina. The choroid fissure closes during week 7, so that the optic stalk, together with the axons of the ganglion cells, forms the **optic nerve (CN II), optic chiasm, and optic tract.** The optic nerve (CN II) is a tract of the diencephalon and has the following characteristics:

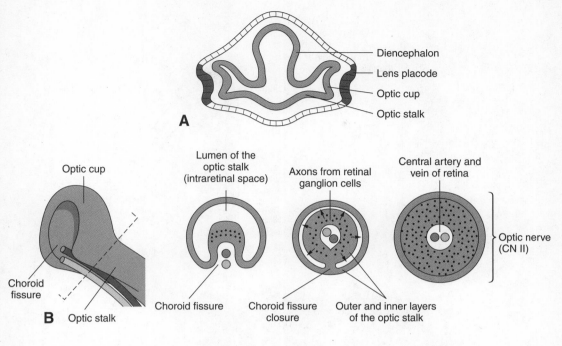

A

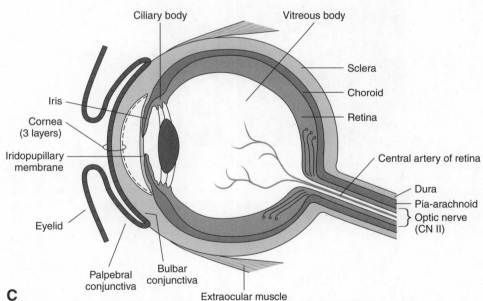

B

C

● **Figure 15.1 (A) The optic cup and optic stalk are evaginations of the diencephalon.** The optic cup induces surface ectoderm to differentiate into the lens placode. **(B) Formation of the optic nerve (CN II) from the optic stalk.** The choroid fissure, which is located on the undersurface of the optic stalk, permits access of the hyaloid artery and vein to the inner aspect of the eye. The choroid fissure eventually closes. As ganglion cells form in the retina, axons accumulate in the optic stalk and cause the inner and outer layers of the optic stalk to fuse, obliterating the lumen (or intraretinal space) and forming the optic nerve. **(C) The adult eye.** Note that the sclera is continuous with the dura mater and the choroid is continuous with the pia-arachnoid. The iridopupillary membrane is normally obliterated.

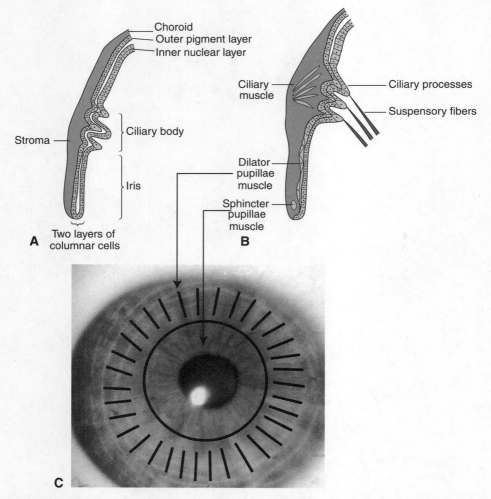

● **Figure 15.2 (A,B) Sagittal sections through the developing iris and ciliary body.** The iris and ciliary body form from the outer pigment layer and inner neural layer of the optic cup. In the adult, this embryological origin is reflected histologically by two layers of columnar epithelium that line both the iris and ciliary body. Note the dilator and sphincter pupillae muscles associated with the iris and the ciliary muscle associated with the ciliary body. **(C) Photograph of the human eye.** Note the radial arrangement (spoke-like pattern) of the dilator pupillae muscle around the entire iris. Note the circular arrangement of the sphincter pupillae muscle around the edge of the entire iris.

1. It is not completely myelinated until 3 months after birth; it is myelinated by oligo-dendrocytes.
2. It is not capable of regeneration after transection.
3. It is invested by the meninges and therefore is surrounded by a subarachnoid space, which plays a role in papilledema.

Development of Other Eye Structures

A. Sclera. The sclera develops from mesoderm surrounding the optic cup. The sclera forms an outer **fibrous** layer that is continuous with the dura mater posteriorly and the cornea anteriorly.

B. Choroid. The choroid develops from mesoderm surrounding the optic cup. The choroid forms a **vascular** layer that is continuous with the pia-arachnoid posteriorly and iris/ciliary body anteriorly.

C. Anterior chamber. The anterior chamber develops from mesoderm over the anterior aspect of the eye that is continuous with the sclera and undergoes vacuolization to form a chamber. The anterior chamber essentially splits the mesoderm into two layers:

1. The mesoderm posterior to the anterior chamber is called the **iridopupillary membrane,** which is normally resorbed prior to birth.

2. The mesoderm anterior to the anterior chamber develops into the **substantia propria of the cornea** and **corneal endothelium.**

D. Cornea. The cornea develops from both surface ectoderm and mesoderm lying anterior to the anterior chamber. The surface ectoderm forms the **anterior epithelium of the cornea.** The mesoderm forms the **substantia propria of the cornea (i.e., Bowman layer, stroma, and Descemet membrane)** and **corneal endothelium.**

E. Lens. The lens develops from surface ectoderm, which forms the **lens placode.** The lens placode invaginates to form the **lens vesicle.** The adult lens is completely surrounded by a **lens capsule.** The **lens epithelium** is a simple cuboidal epithelium located beneath the capsule on the anterior surface only. The lens epithelium is mitotically active and migrates to the equatorial region of the lens. The **lens fibers** are prismatic remnants of the lens epithelium, which lose their nuclei and organelles. The lens fibers are filled with cytoskeletal proteins called **filensin** and **α,β,γ-crystallin,** which maintain the conformation and transparency of the lens.

F. Vitreous body. The vitreous body develops from mesoderm that migrates through the choroid fissure and forms a transparent gelatinous substance between the lens and retina. It contains the **hyaloid artery,** which is later obliterated to form the **hyaloid canal** of the adult eye.

G. Canal of Schlemm. This canal is found at the sclerocorneal junction called the **limbus** and drains the aqueous humor into the venous circulation. An obstruction of the canal of Schlemm results in increased intraocular pressure **(glaucoma).**

H. Extraocular muscles. The extraocular muscles develop from mesoderm of **somitomeres 1, 2, and 3** (also called preoptic myotomes) that surround the optic cup.

TABLE 15-1	EMBRYONIC EYE STRUCTURES AND THEIR ADULT DERIVATIVES
Embryonic Structure	**Adult Derivative**
Diencephalon (neuroectoderm)	
Optic cup	Retina, iris epithelium, dilator and sphincter pupillae muscles of iris, ciliary body epithelium
Optic stalk	Optic nerve (CN II), optic chiasm, optic tract
Surface ectoderm	Lens, anterior epithelium of cornea, bulbar and palpebral conjunctiva
Mesoderm	Sclera, choroid, stroma of iris, stroma of ciliary body, ciliary muscle, substantia propria of cornea, corneal endothelium, vitreous body, central artery and vein of retina, extraocular muscles

Congenital Malformations of the Eye (Figure 15-3)

A. **Coloboma iridis** is a cleft in the iris caused by failure of the choroid fissure to close in week 7 of development; it may extend into the ciliary body, retina, choroid, or optic nerve. A **palpebral coloboma,** a notch in the eyelid, results from a defect in the developing eyelid.

B. **Congenital cataracts** are opacities of the lens and are usually bilateral. They are fairly common and may result from the following: rubella virus infection, toxoplasmosis, congenital syphilis, Down syndrome (trisomy 21), or galactosemia (an inborn error of metabolism).

C. **Congenital glaucoma (buphthalmos)** is increased intraocular pressure due to abnormal development of the canal of Schlemm or the iridocorneal filtration angle. It is usually genetically determined but may result from maternal rubella infection.

D. **Detached retina** may result from head trauma or may be congenital. The site of detachment is between the outer and inner layers of the optic cup (i.e., between the retinal pigment epithelial layer and outer segment layer of rods and cones of the neural retina).

E. **Persistent iridopupillary membrane** consists of strands of connective tissue that partially cover the pupil; however, it seldom affects vision.

F. **Microphthalmia** is a small eye, usually associated with intrauterine infections from the TORCH group of microorganisms (*Toxoplasma,* **r**ubella virus, **c**ytomegalovirus, and **h**erpes simplex virus).

G. **Anophthalmia** is absence of the eye. It is due to failure of the optic vesicle to form.

H. **Cyclopia** is a single orbit and one eye. It is due to failure of median cerebral structures to develop.

I. **Retinocele** results from herniation of the retina into the sclera or from failure of the choroid fissure to close.

J. **Retrolental fibroplasia** (retinopathy of prematurity) is an oxygen-induced retinopathy seen in premature infants.

K. **Papilledema** is edema of the optic disk (papilla) due to increased intracranial pressure. This pressure is reflected into the subarachnoid space, which surrounds the optic nerve (CN II).

L. **Retinitis pigmentosa (RP)** is a hereditary degeneration and atrophy of the retina. RP may be transmitted as an autosomal recessive, autosomal dominant, or X-linked trait. It is characterized by a degeneration of the rods, night blindness (nyctalopia), and "gun barrel vision." RP may also be due to abetalipoproteinemia (Bassen-Kornzweig syndrome), which can be arrested with massive doses of vitamin A.

M. **Retinoblastoma (RB)** is a tumor of the retina that occurs in childhood and develops from precursor cells in the immature retina. The RB gene is located on chromosome 13 and encodes for RB protein, which binds to a gene-regulatory protein and causes suppression of the cell cycle (i.e., the RB gene is a **tumor-suppressor gene,** also called an **antioncogene**). A mutation in the RB gene will encode an abnormal RB protein such that there is no suppression of the cell cycle. This leads to the formation of RB. Hereditary RB causes multiple tumors in both eyes. Nonhereditary RB causes one tumor in one eye.

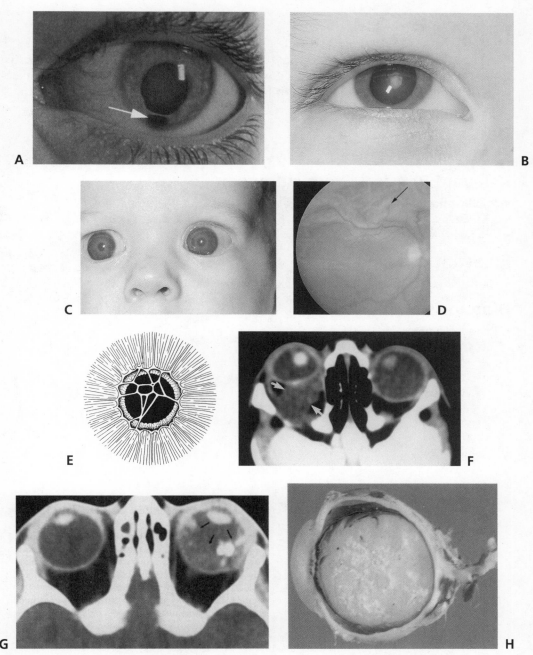

● **Figure 15.3 (A) Coloboma iridis.** Note the cleft in the iris (black spot at arrow). **(B) Congenital cataracts.** Note the lens opacity, indicating a polar cataract. Lens opacities in infants may be isolated or associated with a systemic condition. The morphology of infantile cataracts is distinctive, which differentiates infantile cataracts from other forms of cataracts. The location of the opacity in the eye of the infant permits a classification of polar, zonular (lamellar), nuclear, sutural, or total. **(C) Congenital glaucoma (buphthalmos).** Note the enlarged right and left eyes. The dot reflex from the flash camera is not sharp. An enlarged eye is suspected when the corneal diameter exceeds 11 mm in a term newborn. If the eye is enlarged, infantile glaucoma caused by elevated intraocular pressure should be suspected immediately. Infantile glaucoma may also present with tearing, squinting, photosensitivity, and a cloudy cornea. The cornea often has horizontal lines, called Haab striae, which result from a disruption of the Descemet membrane. **(D) Detached retina.** Note the rough, corrugated, opaque appearance of the detached retina (arrow). **(E) Persistent iridopupillary membrane.** Note the strands of connective tissue partially covering the pupil. **(F) Microphthalmia.** CT scan shows exophthalmos, small right globe, and a retro-ocular mass (arrows). **(G) Retinoblastoma.** CT scan shows multiple tumor calcifications (arrows) within the left intraorbital mass. **(H) Photograph shows a large retinoblastoma that fills the entire eye.**

Case Study

A young mother brings in her 3-year-old son because of "a white spot in his eye." She first noticed the spot in a photograph taken 2 weeks earlier. She remembers hearing about another family member with the same sort of spot who eventually went blind. What is the most likely diagnosis?

Differentials

- Congenital cataract, congenital glaucoma, retinoblastoma

Relevant Physical Exam Findings

- Pupil with white spots
- Poor vision
- Crossed eyes

Relevant Lab Findings

- Genetic testing shows a mutation of the RB gene on chromosome 13.

Diagnosis

- Retinoblastoma

Chapter 16

Body Cavities

I **Formation of the Intraembryonic Coelom** **(Figure 16-1).** The formation of the intraembryonic coelom begins when spaces coalesce within the lateral mesoderm and form a horseshoe-shaped space that opens into the chorionic cavity (extraembryonic coelom) on the right and left side. The intraembryonic coelom is remodeled due to the craniocaudal folding and lateral folding of the embryo. The intraembryonic coelom can best be visualized as a balloon whose walls are visceral mesoderm (closest to the viscera) and somatic mesoderm (closest to the body wall). The intraembryonic coelom provides the needed room for the growth of various organs.

II **Partitioning of the Intraembryonic Coelom.** The intraembryonic coelom is initially one continuous space. In order to form the definitive adult pericardial, pleural, and peritoneal cavities, two partitions must develop. These two partitions are the **paired pleuropericardial membranes** and the **diaphragm.**

A. The **paired pleuropericardial membranes** (Figure 16-1) are sheets of somatic mesoderm that separate the **pericardial cavity** from the **pleural cavities.** The formation of these membranes appears to be aided by lung buds invading the lateral body wall and by tension on the common cardinal veins resulting from rapid longitudinal growth.

These membranes develop into the definitive **fibrous pericardium** surrounding the heart.

B. The **diaphragm** (Figure 16-1) separates the **pleural cavities** from the **peritoneal cavity.** The diaphragm is formed through the fusion of tissue from four different sources:

1. The **septum transversum**—a thick mass of mesoderm located between the primitive heart tube and the developing liver. The septum transversum is the primordium of the **central tendon of the diaphragm** in the adult.

2. The **paired pleuroperitoneal membranes**—sheets of somatic mesoderm that appear to develop from the dorsal and dorsolateral body wall by an unknown mechanism.

3. The **dorsal mesentery of the esophagus,** which is invaded by myoblasts and forms the **crura of the diaphragm** in the adult.

4. The **body wall,** which contributes muscle to the peripheral portions of the definitive diaphragm.

III **Positional Changes of the Diaphragm.** During week 4 of development, the diaphragm becomes innervated by the **phrenic nerves,** which originate from C3, C4, and C5 and pass through the pleuropericardial membranes (this explains the definitive location of the phrenic nerves associated with the fibrous pericardium). By week 8, there is an apparent **descent of the diaphragm to L1** because of the rapid growth of the neural tube. The phrenic nerves are carried along with the "descending diaphragm," which explains their unusually great length in the adult.

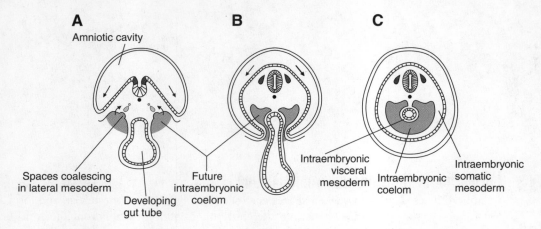

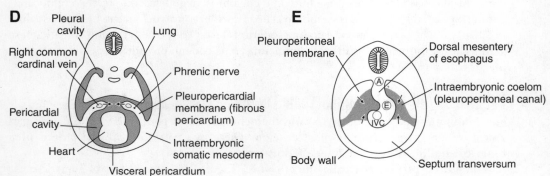

● **Figure 16.1 Diagrams illustrating the formation and partitioning of the intraembryonic coelom (IC).**
(A–C) Cross sections show various stages of IC formation while the embryo undergoes lateral folding. **(D)** Cross section shows two folds of intraembryonic somatic mesoderm carrying the phrenic nerves and common cardinal veins. The two folds fuse in the midline (arrows) to form the pleuropericardial membrane. This separates the pericardial cavity (shaded) from the pleural cavity (shaded). **(E)** Cross section of an embryo at week 5 shows the four components that fuse (arrows) to form the diaphragm, which closes off the IC between the pleural and peritoneal cavities. The portions of the IC that connect the pleural and pericardial cavities in the embryo are called the pleuroperitoneal canals (shaded). A = aorta, E = esophagus, IVC = inferior vena cava.

 Clinical Considerations (Figure 16-2)

    A. Congenital diaphragmatic hernia is a herniation of abdominal contents into the pleural cavity caused by a **failure of the pleuroperitoneal membrane** to develop or fuse with the other components of the diaphragm. A congenital diaphragmatic hernia is most commonly found on the **left posterolateral side** and is usually life-threatening, because abdominal contents compress the lung buds, causing **pulmonary hypoplasia.** Clinical signs in the newborn include an unusually flat abdomen, breathlessness, severe dyspnea, peristaltic bowel sounds over the left chest, and cyanosis. This hernia can be detected prenatally by ultrasonography.

    B. Esophageal hiatal hernia is a herniation of the stomach through the esophageal hiatus into the pleural cavity; it is caused by an abnormally large esophageal hiatus. An esophageal hiatal hernia renders the **esophagogastric sphincter** incompetent, so that stomach contents reflux into the esophagus. Clinical signs in the newborn include vomiting (frequently projectile) when the infant is laid on its back after feeding.

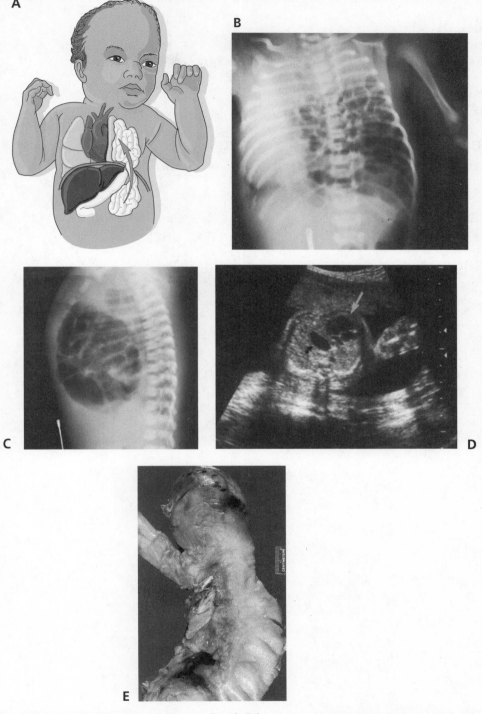

● **Figure 16.2 Congenital diaphragmatic hernia (A–D). (A)** A diagram of a congenital diaphragmatic hernia showing the herniation of intestinal loops into the left pleural cavity (arrow). **(B)** AP radiograph of a congenital diaphragmatic hernia. Note the loops of intestine within the pleural cavity, as indicated by the bowel gas above and below the diaphragm and the mediastinal shift to the right. **(C)** A lateral radiograph of a congenital diaphragmatic hernia. Note the loops of intestine within the pleural cavity, as indicated by the bowel gas above and below the diaphragm. **(D)** A sonogram of a congenital diaphragmatic hernia. Note the heart (white arrow) shifted to the right by a herniated fluid-filled stomach (black arrow). **(E) Photograph of an esophageal hiatal hernia.** Note the large saccular, discolored, ischemic portion of the stomach (arrow) and the deviation of the esophagus to the right.

Case Study

The father of a 1-month-old daughter complains that she frequently "throws up after she eats," and "it just shoots across the room." What is the most likely diagnosis?

Differentials

- Pyloric stenosis, GERD, esophageal hiatal hernia, congenital diaphragmatic hernia

Relevant Physical Exam Findings

- Projectile vomiting after infant is laid on its back after a feeding

Relevant Lab Findings

- Chest radiograph shows herniation of the stomach through the esophageal hiatus into the pleural cavity.

Diagnosis

- Esophageal hiatal hernia

Chapter 17

Integumentary System

Skin. The skin consists of two layers: the outer layer (or **epidermis**) and the deeper connective tissue layer (or **dermis**). Skin functions as a barrier against infection, provides for thermoregulation, and protects the body against dehydration.

A. **Epidermis.** The epidermis is derived from the ectoderm.

1. **Early development.** Initially, the epidermis consists of a single layer of ectodermal cells that give rise to an overlying **periderm** layer. The epidermis soon becomes a three-layered structure consisting of the **stratum basale** (mitotically active), **intermediate layer** (progeny of stratum basale), and the **periderm.** Peridermal cells are eventually desquamated and form part of the **vernix caseosa,** a greasy substance of peridermal cells and sebum from the sebaceous glands, which protects the embryo's skin.

2. **Later development.** The definitive adult layers are formed through the inductive influence of the dermis. The ectodermal cells give rise to five cell layers:
   a. **Stratum basale (stratum germinativum)**
   b. **Stratum spinosum**
   c. **Stratum lucidum**
   d. **Stratum granulosum**
   e. **Stratum corneum.** This layer is associated with the expression of a **56-kda keratin, a 67-kda keratin,** and **filaggrin** (a binding protein).

3. **Other cells of the epidermis**
   a. **Melanoblasts** are derived from **neural crest cells** that migrate into the stratum basale of the epidermis. They differentiate into melanocytes by midpregnancy, when pigment granules called **melanosomes** are observed.
   b. **Langerhans cells** are derived from the **bone marrow (mesoderm)** and migrate into the epidermis. They are involved in antigen presentation.
   c. **Merkel cells** are of uncertain origin. They are associated with free nerve endings and probably function as mechanoreceptors.

B. **Dermis.** The dermis is derived from both the somatic mesoderm located just beneath the ectoderm and the mesoderm of the body's dermatomes. In the head and neck region, the dermis is derived from neural crest cells.

1. **Early development.** The dermis is initially composed of loosely aggregated mesodermal cells frequently referred to as **mesenchymal cells** (or **mesenchyme**). The mesenchymal cells secrete a watery-type extracellular matrix rich in glycogen and hyaluronic acid.

2. **Later development.** The mesenchymal cells differentiate into fibroblasts, which secrete increasing amounts of collagen and elastic fibers into the extracellular matrix. Vascularization occurs. Sensory nerves grow into the dermis. The dermis forms projections into the epidermis called **dermal papillae,** which contain tactile sensory receptors (e.g., Meissner's corpuscles).

C. Clinical correlations (Figure 17-1)

1. Oculocutaneous albinism (OCA)

a. **Type I OCA (tyrosinase-negative; classic type)** is an autosomal recessive disorder in which melanocytes **fail to produce melanin pigment.** The cause is a complete absence of the enzyme **tyrosinase** due to mutations in both copies of the tyrosinase gene, located on **chromosome 11q14-q21.** These individuals have pink skin, gray-blue eyes, and white hair at birth and throughout life. Type I OCA is also associated with **Chediak-Higashi syndrome** (an autosomal recessive disorder) characterized by neutropenia, albinism, cranial/peripheral neuropathy, and a tendency to develop repeated infections.

b. **Type II OCA (tyrosinase-positive)** is an autosomal recessive disorder in which melanocytes **produce some melanin pigment.** The cause is a complete absence of the **P protein** (localizes to the melanosome membrane; function unknown) due to mutations in both copies of the *P* gene, located on **chromosome 15q11-13.** These individuals have pink skin, gray-blue eyes, and dark hair at birth, but the pigment of the skin, eyes, and hair increases as the patient ages.

c. **Piebaldism,** an autosomal dominant disorder, is a localized albinism in which there is a lack of melanin in isolated patches of skin and/or hair. In general, albinism predisposes to basal cell carcinoma, squamous cell carcinoma, and malignant melanoma.

2. Ichthyosis is excessive keratinization of the skin, which is characterized by dryness, scaling, and cracks, which may form deep fissures. In severe cases, a **harlequin fetus** may result. This condition is usually inherited as an autosomal recessive trait but may also be X-linked.

3. Psoriasis is a skin disease characterized by **excessive cell proliferation** in the stratum basale and the stratum spinosum. This results in thickening of the epidermis and a shorter regeneration time of the epidermis.

4. Ehlers-Danlos syndrome is an autosomal dominant genetic disorder involving the gene for **peptidyl lysine hydroxylase,** an enzyme necessary for the hydroxylation of lysine residues of collagen. It affects mainly type I and type III collagen. This syndrome is characterized by extremely stretchable and fragile skin, hypermobile joints, aneurysms of blood vessels, and rupture of the bowel.

5. Angiomas are common cutaneous vascular malformations—that is, benign tumors of endothelial cells. The major groups seen in children are involuting and noninvoluting lesions. These may be flat (i.e., macular or telangiectatic) or raised (i.e., hemangiomatous).

a. A **superficial strawberry hemangioma (involuting)** is a raised lesion that is usually bright red or purplish red with well-defined margins. This lesion appears a few days or weeks after birth as a pink or red macule and enlarges during the first 5–6 months. This lesion is a firm, rubbery mass that compresses minimally and blanches incompletely with pressure.

b. A **deep cavernous hemangioma (involuting)** is a raised lesion (it arises deeper in the dermis) that usually imparts a reddish blue color to the overlying skin; it has poorly defined margins. This lesion is a cystic, "bag of worms" mass that compresses to half of its size with pressure and then resumes its usual size.

c. A **port-wine nevus or nevus flammeus** (noninvoluting) is a flat lesion that is usually dark red or bluish with well-defined margins. This lesion shows stable growth with the child and blanches minimally with pressure. It produces "birthmarks" on the skin. A port-wine stain is a birthmark covering the area of distribution of the trigeminal nerve (CN V); it is frequently associated with a hemangioma of the meninges called **Sturge-Weber syndrome.**

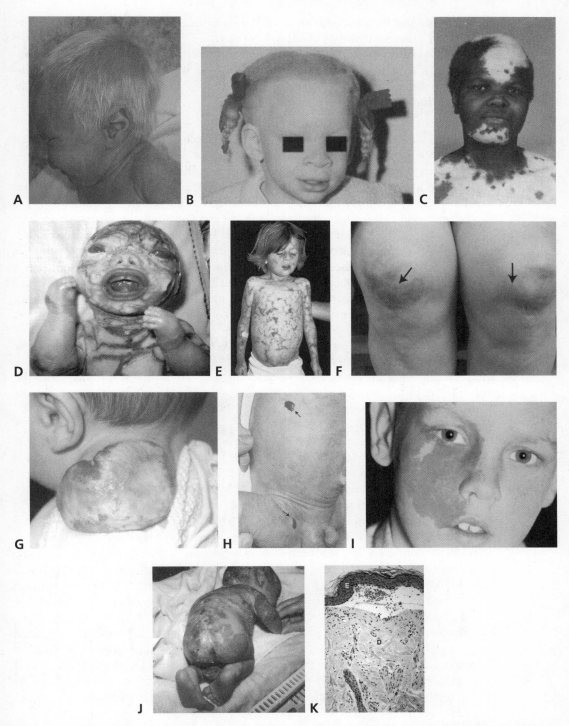

● **Figure 17.1 (A) Type I oculocutaneous albinism (OCA). (B) Type II OCA in a black female child. (C) Piebald-ism in a black female child. (D) Harlequin fetus. (E,F) Ehlers-Danlos syndrome. (E)** Ehlers-Danlos type IV (ecchy-motic variant) is associated with thin skin and visible veins. In other types the skin is extremely stretchable. **(F)** Note the cigarette-paper scars over the knees (arrows). **(G) Superficial strawberry hemangioma. (H) Deep cavernous he-mangioma.** Note the hemangiomas (arrows). **(I) Port-wine nevus or nevus flammeus.** This birthmark darkens with exertion or temperature exposure. Unlike a hemangioma, this birthmark does not fade with time. **(J,K) Epidermolysis bullosa in a young infant, with widespread bullae (blisters) and erosion of the skin.** LM shows a pathological cleft (*) between the epidermis (E) and dermis (D). There is also some scarring in the dermis.

6. **Junctional epidermolysis bullosa (JEB)** comprises a group of autosomal recessive disorders characterized by bulla (blister) formation. The cause is a mutation in the gene for **laminin 5,** which alters adhesion of stratum basale to the basement membrane. The epidermis is intact but is separated from the underlying dermis. This disease is usually fatal by 3-4 years of age because of the associated hypoproteinemia, anemia, and infection.

Ⅱ Hair and Nails.   Hair and nails are derived from the ectoderm.

A. Hair. At week 12, cells from the stratum basale grow into the underlying dermis and form the **hair follicle.** The deepest part of the hair follicle soon becomes club-shaped, forming the **hair bulb.** The hair bulbs are invaginated by mesoderm, called the **hair papillae,** which are rapidly infiltrated by blood vessels and nerve endings.

The epithelial cells within the hair bulb differentiate into the **germinal matrix,** where cells proliferate, grow toward the surface, keratinize, and form the **hair shaft.** These cells also form the **internal root sheath.** Other epithelial cells of the hair follicle form the **external root sheath,** which is continuous with the epidermis and has a prominent subjacent basement membrane called the **glassy membrane.** Mesodermal cells of the dermis that surround the invaginating hair follicle form the **dermal root sheath** and the **arrector pili muscle.** The first fine hairs, called **lanugo hairs,** are sloughed off at birth.

BMP-2 (bone morphogenetic protein), **FGF-2** (fibroblast growth factor), **sonic hedgehog,** and **Msx** (a homeobox gene) appear to be important in hair development.

B. Nails develop from the epidermis. The nails first develop on the tips of the digits and then migrate to the dorsal surface, taking their innervation with them; this is why the median nerve innervates the dorsal surface of 3 1/2 digits (I–IV).

C. Clinical correlations

1. **Alopecia** is baldness resulting from an absence or faulty development of the hair follicles.
2. **Hypertrichosis** is an overgrowth of hair. It is frequently associated with spina bifida occulta, which is seen as a patch of hair overlying the defect.
3. **Pili torti** is a familial disorder characterized by **twisted hairs.** It is seen in **Menkes (kinky-hair) disease,** an X-linked recessive neurologic disorder involving a defect in intestinal copper transport.
4. **Trichorrhexis nodosa** is **brittle hair** that breaks easily and is usually associated with metabolic conditions like **argininosuccinic aciduria,** an autosomal recessive genetic disorder that causes a deficiency in the enzyme argininosuccinase of the urea cycle.
5. **Beaded hair** is characterized by elliptical nodes along the hair, which breaks easily at the internodes; it is usually associated with **monilethrix.** Monilethrix is an autosomal dominant genetic disorder.
6. **Trichothiodystrophy** is a very rare autosomal recessive genetic disorder characterized by short, brittle hair with alternating light and dark bands called **"tiger-tail" hair.**
7. **Uncombable hair syndrome ("spun-glass" hair)** is an autosomal dominant genetic disorder characterized by blonde, dry, shiny hair that cannot be combed into place. The hair is a triangular in diameter with a canal-like groove called pili trianguli et canaliculi.

Ⅲ Mammary, Sweat, and Sebaceous Glands are all derived from the surface ectoderm.

A. Mammary glands develop from the **mammary ridge,** a downgrowth of the epidermis (ectoderm) into the underlying dermis (mesoderm). Canalization of these epithelial downgrowths results in the formation of **alveoli** and **lactiferous ducts.** The lactiferous ducts drain into an epithelial pit, the future **nipple.**

B. **Eccrine** and **apocrine sweat glands** develop from downgrowths of the epidermis into the underlying dermis.

C. **Sebaceous glands** develop from the epithelial wall of the hair follicle and elaborate **sebum** into the hair follicles. The tarsal (meibomian) glands of the eyelids do not communicate with hair follicles.

D. **Clinical correlations (Figure 17-2)**

1. **Gynecomastia** is a condition in which there is excessive development of the male mammary glands. It is frequently associated with Klinefelter syndrome (47, XXY).
2. **Breast hypertrophy** may occur early in infancy.
3. **Breast hypoplasia** generally occurs asymmetrically when one breast fails to develop completely.
4. **Polythelia** is a condition in which supernumerary nipples occur along the mammary ridge.
5. **Polymastia** is a condition in which supernumerary breasts occur along the mammary ridge.

 Teeth (Figure 17-3) develop from ectoderm and an underlying layer of neural crest cells.

A. The **dental lamina** develops from the oral epithelium (ectoderm) as a downgrowth into the underlying neural crest layer. The dental lamina gives rise to **tooth buds,** which develop into the **enamel organs.**

B. The **enamel organs** are derived from ectoderm and develop first for the 20 deciduous teeth, then for the 32 permanent teeth. The enamel organs give rise to **ameloblasts,** which produce **enamel.**

C. The **dental papillae** are formed by neural crest cells underlying the enamel organs. The dental papillae give rise to the **odontoblasts** (which produce **predentin** and **dentin**) and **dental pulp.**

D. The **dental sacs** are formed by the condensation of neural crest cells around the dental papillae. The dental sacs give rise to **cementoblasts** (which produce **cementum**) and the **periodontal ligaments.**

E. **Clinical correlations**

1. **Defective enamel formation (amelogenesis imperfecta)** is an autosomal dominant trait.
2. **Defective dentin formation (dentinogenesis imperfecta)** is an autosomal dominant trait.
3. **Vitamin A deficiency.** If this deficiency is severe, ameloblast cells will atrophy, which results in the absence of enamel. In less severe cases, there is **enamel hypoplasia.**
4. **Vitamin D deficiency.** A severe vitamin D deficiency in children results in rickets, a condition characterized by insufficient deposition of calcium in bony tissue. In teeth, vitamin D deficiency causes **enamel and dentin hypoplasia.**
5. **Tetracycline discoloration.** If tetracycline antibiotics are administered to a pregnant woman, permanent **brown-gray staining** of the teeth will result in the child. Tetracycline is deposited in bone and teeth during mineralization.

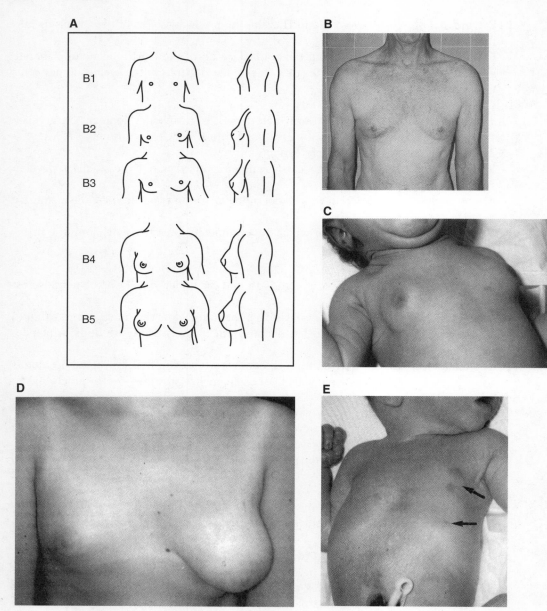

● **Figure 17.2 (A) The Tanner stages of breast development are guidelines in assessing whether a female adolescent is developing normally.** In stage B1 (preadolescent), there is elevation of the papilla only. In stage B2 (breast bud stage), there is elevation of the breast and papilla as a small mound and enlargement of the areolar diameter. In stage B3, there is further enlargement of the breast and areola with no separation of their contours. In stage B4, there is further enlargement with projection of the areola and papilla to form a secondary mound above the level of the breast. In stage B5 (mature stage), there is projection of the papilla only due to a recession of the areola to the general contour of the breast. **(B) Gynecomastia in a male. (C) Breast hypertrophy in a 1-month-old female infant. (D) Breast hypoplasia of the right breast in a 16-year-old female. (E) Polythelia is shown, where two rudimentary nipples (arrows) are located along the left mammary line.**

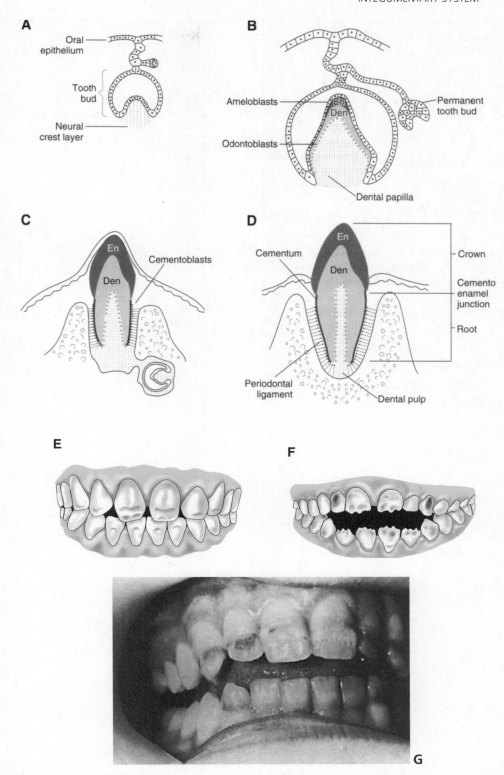

● **Figure 17.3 (A–D) Diagram of successive stages in the development of a tooth. (A)** At week 8. **(B)** At week 28. Note the formation of enamel (En) by ameloblasts and dentin (Den) by odontoblasts. **(C)** At month 6 postnatal. Note the early tooth eruption. **(D)** At month 18 postnatal. Note the fully erupted deciduous tooth. Ameloblasts are no longer present, which means that further enamel formation is not possible. **(E) Clinical appearance of teeth in vitamin A deficiency. (F) Clinical appearance of teeth in vitamin D deficiency. (G) Clinical appearance of teeth in tetracycline staining.**

Case Study

A father brings his 8-year-old son to the clinic and tells you that the child "is bleeding a lot" and that he "comes in from playing with a lot of bruises." The son tells you that he is "one of the coolest kids in school" because "he can pull his skin out all over the place." Then he proceeds to demonstrate this fact by pulling his ears out several inches away from his body. What is the most likely diagnosis?

Differentials

• Marfan syndrome, Ehlers-Danlos syndrome, osteogenesis imperfecta

Relevant Physical Exam Findings

• Highly elastic velvety skin
• Fragile skin that bruises easily
• Loose, unstable, hyperextensible joints
• Bleeding from fragile blood vessels

Relevant Lab Findings

• Testing shows a defect in the gene for peptidyl lysine hydroxylase.

Diagnosis

• Ehlers-Danlos syndrome

Chapter 18

Skeletal System

Skull (**Figure 18-1**). The skull can be divided into two parts: the neurocranium and viscerocranium.

A. Neurocranium. The neurocranium consists of the flat bones of the skull (cranial vault) and the base of the skull. The neurocranium develops from neural crest cells except for the basilar part of the occipital bone, which forms from mesoderm of the occipital sclerotomes.

B. Viscerocranium. The viscerocranium consists of the bones of the face involving the pharyngeal arches. The viscerocranium develops from neural crest cells except for the laryngeal cartilage, which forms from mesoderm within pharyngeal arches 4 and 6.

C. Sutures

1. During fetal life and infancy, the flat bones of the skull are separated by dense connective tissue (fibrous joints) called **sutures.** There are five sutures: the **frontal suture, sagittal suture, lambdoid suture, coronal suture,** and **squamous suture.**

2. Sutures allow the flat bones of the skull to deform during childbirth (called **molding**) and expand during childhood as the brain grows. Molding may exert considerable tension at the "obstetrical hinge" (junction of the squamous and lateral parts of the occipital bone), such that the **great cerebral vein (of Galen)** is ruptured during childbirth.

D. Fontanelles are large fibrous areas where several sutures meet. There are six fontanelles: the **anterior fontanelle, posterior fontanelle, two sphenoid fontanelles,** and **two mastoid fontanelles.**

1. The anterior fontanelle is the largest fontanelle and readily palpable in the infant. It pulsates because of the underlying cerebral arteries and can be used to obtain a blood sample from the underlying **superior sagittal sinus.**

2. The **anterior fontanelle and the mastoid fontanelles** close at about **2 years of age,** when the main growth of the brain ceases.

3. The **posterior fontanelle and sphenoid fontanelles** close at about **6 months of age.**

E. Clinical correlations

1. **Abnormalities in skull shape** may result from failure of cranial sutures to form or from premature closure of sutures (**craniosynostoses**).

   a. **Microcephaly** results from failure of the brain to grow; usually associated with mental retardation.

   b. **Oxycephaly (turricephaly or acrocephaly)** is a **tower-like skull** caused by premature closure of the **lambdoid and coronal sutures.** It should be differentiated from **Crouzon syndrome,** which is a dominant genetic condition with a presentation quite similar to that of oxycephaly but is accompanied by malformations of the face, teeth, and ears.

   c. **Plagiocephaly** is an asymmetric skull caused by premature closure of the **lambdoid and coronal sutures** on one side of the skull.

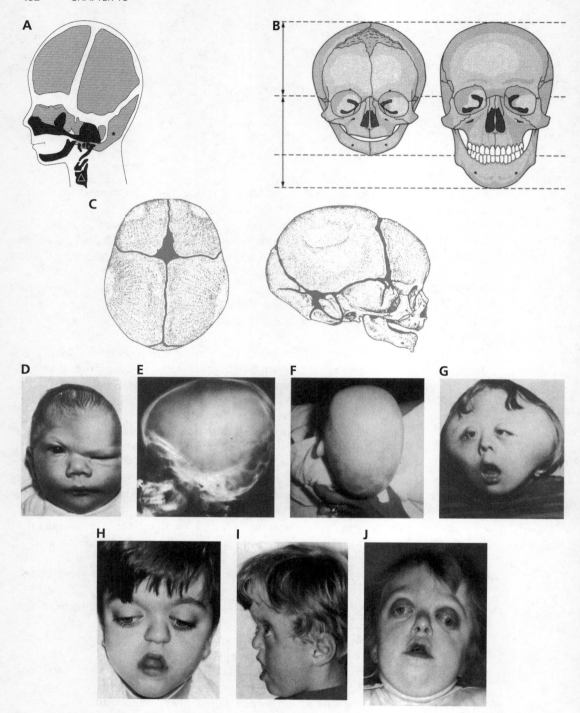

● **Figure 18.1 (A) A diagram of the newborn skull indicating the neurocranium (shaded area) and the viscero-cranium (black area).** The bones of the neurocranium and viscerocranium are derived almost entirely from neural crest cells except for the basilar part of the occipital bone (*), which forms from mesoderm of the occipital sclerotomes, and the laryngeal cartilages (▲), which form from mesoderm within pharyngeal arches 4 and 6. **(B) A diagram depicting the postnatal growth of the skull.** After birth, the skull continues ossification toward the sutures. However, the face is relatively underdeveloped and undergoes dramatic changes during childhood and adolescence with the eruption of teeth, formation of sinuses, and elongation of the maxilla and mandible. Note that the profound postnatal changes of the skull are due to the development of the viscerocranium. **(C) Diagram of the sutures and fontanelles.** F = frontal suture, C = coronal suture, SS = sagittal suture, L = lambdoid suture, Sq = squamous suture, AF = anterior fontanelle, PF = posterior fontanelle, MF = mastoid fontanelle, SF = sphenoid fontanelle. **(D) Plagiocephaly. (E) Brachiocephaly. (F) Scapho-cephaly. (G) Kleeblattschädel. (H) Crouzon syndrome. (I) Apert syndrome. (J) Pfeiffer syndrome.**

d. **Brachycephaly** is a short, square-shaped skull caused by premature closure of the **coronal sutures.**

e. **Scaphocephaly** is a long skull (in the AP plane) caused by premature closure of the **sagittal suture.**

f. **Kleeblattschädel** is a cloverleaf skull caused by premature closure of **all sutures,** forcing the brain growth through the anterior and sphenoid fontanelles.

g. **Crouzon syndrome** is an autosomal dominant genetic disorder characterized by premature craniosynostosis, midface hypoplasia with shallow orbits, and ocular proptosis. This syndrome is caused by a mutation in the gene for fibroblast growth factor receptor 2 (FGFR2), located on chromosome 10q25-q26.

h. **Apert syndrome** is an autosomal dominant genetic disorder characterized by craniosynostosis leading to turribrachycephaly; syndactyly of hands and feet; various ankyloses; progressive synostoses of the hands, feet, and cervical spine; and mental retardation. This syndrome is caused by a mutation in the gene for fibroblast growth factor receptor 2 (FGFR2) located on chromosome 10q25-q26, which is exclusively of paternal origin.

i. **Pfeiffer syndrome** is an autosomal dominant genetic disorder characterized by craniosynostosis leading to turribrachycephaly, syndactyly of hands and feet, and broad thumbs and great toes. This syndrome is caused by a mutation in the gene for fibroblast growth factor receptor 2 (FGFR2) located on chromosome 10q25-q26.

2. **Temporal bone formation**

a. **Mastoid process.** This portion of the temporal bone is absent at birth, which leaves the **facial nerve (CN VII)** relatively unprotected as it emerges from the stylomastoid foramen. In a difficult delivery, forceps may damage CN VII. The mastoid process forms by 2 years of age.

b. **Petrosquamous fissure.** The petrous and squamous portions of the temporal bone are separated by the petrosquamous fissure, which opens directly into the mastoid antrum of the middle ear. This fissure, which may remain open until 20 years of age, provides a route for the spread of infection from the middle ear to the meninges.

3. The **sphenoccipital joint** is a site of growth up to about 20 years of age.

Ⅱ Vertebral Column (Figure 18-2)

A. **Vertebrae in general.** Mesodermal cells from the sclerotome migrate and condense around the notochord to form the **centrum,** around the neural tube to form the **vertebral arches,** and in the body wall to form the **costal processes.**

1. The centrum forms the **vertebral body.**

2. The vertebral arches form the **pedicles, laminae, spinous process, articular processes**, and the **transverse processes.**

3. The costal processes form the **ribs.**

B. The **atlas (C1) and axis (C2)** are highly modified vertebrae.

1. The atlas has no vertebral body or spinous process.

2. The axis has an **odontoid process (dens),** which represents the vertebral body of the atlas.

C. The **sacrum** is a large triangular fusion of five sacral vertebrae forming the posterosuperior wall of the pelvic cavity.

D. The **coccyx** is a small triangular fusion of four rudimentary vertebrae.

E. The **intersegmental position of vertebrae**

1. As mesodermal cells from the sclerotome migrate toward the notochord and neural tube, they split into a **cranial portion** and a **caudal portion.** The caudal portion of each sclerotome fuses with the cranial portion of the succeeding sclerotome, which results in the intersegmental position of the vertebrae. The splitting of the sclerotome is important because it allows the developing spinal nerve a route of access to the myotomes, which it must innervate.

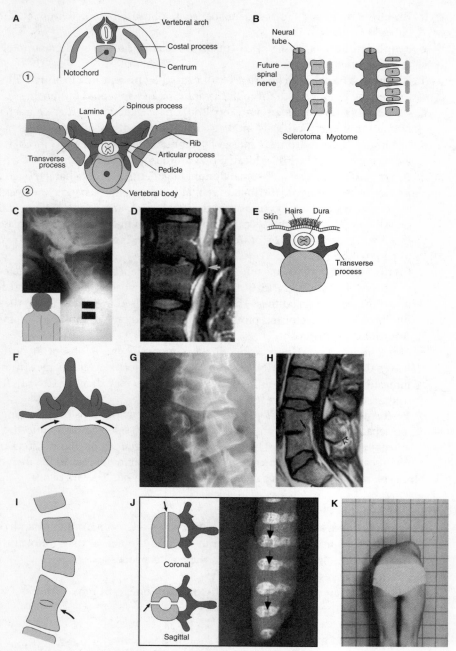

● **Figure 18.2 (A) Diagram indicating the development of a typical thoracic vertebra.** (1) At about 5–7 weeks. Mesodermal cells from the sclerotome demonstrate three distinct condensations: centrum, vertebral arch, and costal process. At birth, three ossification centers are present: one in the centrum and one in each vertebral arch. From 3–5 years of age, the vertebral arches fuse with each other and the centrum. Ossification ends at about 25 years of age. (2) Adult. Each condensation develops into distinct components of the adult vertebrae, as indicated by the shading. **(B) Diagram depicting the splitting of the sclerotome (S) into caudal and cranial portions as the spinal nerves grow out to innervate the myotome (M).** The dotted lines indicate where the sclerotome splits, thus allowing the growing spinal nerve to reach the myotome. **(C) Congenital brevicollis.** Radiograph shows congenital fusion of cervical vertebrae. **(D) Intervertebral disk herniation.** MRI shows the protrusion of the L2 disk, causing extradural compression of cauda equina nerve roots (arrow). **(E) Spina bifida occulta. (F) Spondylolisthesis.** Arrows indicate the congenital absence of the pedicles. **(G) Hemivertebrae.** Radiograph indicates a hemivertebra. **(H) Vertebral bar.** MRI shows partial fusion (solid arrow) of the L4-L5 vertebral bodies posteriorly. Note also the single fused spinous process (open arrow). **(I) Block vertebra. (J) Coronal and sagittal cleft vertebrae.** Radiograph shows coronal clefts in vertebrae L1, L2, and L4 (arrow). **(K) Scoliosis.** The forward-bending examination will detect even very small curvatures. The prominence (arrow) is produced by chest wall asymmetry.

2. In the cervical region, the caudal portion of the fourth occipital sclerotome (O4) fuses with cranial portion of the first cervical (C1) sclerotome to form the base of the occipital bone, which allows C1 spinal nerve to exit between the base of the occipital bone and the C1 vertebrae.

F. Curves

1. The **primary curves** are the **thoracic** and **sacral curvatures,** which form during the fetal period.

2. **The secondary curves** are the **cervical** and **lumbar curvatures,** which form after birth as a result of lifting the head and walking, respectively.

G. Joints of the vertebral column

1. Synovial joints

a. The **atlanto-occipital joint** lies between C1 (atlas) and the occipital condyles.

b. The **atlantoaxial joint** lies between C1 (atlas) and C2 (axis).

c. **Facets (zygapophyseal)** are joints between the inferior and superior articular facets.

2. Secondary cartilaginous joints (symphyses) are the joints between the vertebral bodies, in which the **intervertebral disks** play a role. An intervertebral disk consists of:

a. The **nucleus pulposus.** This is a remnant of the embryonic **notochord.** By 20 years of age, all notochordal cells have degenerated, such that all notochordal vestiges in the adult are limited to just a noncellular matrix.

b. The **annulus fibrosus.** This is an outer rim of fibrocartilage derived from mesoderm found between the vertebral bodies.

H. Clinical correlations

1. Congenital brevicollis (Klippel-Feil syndrome) results from fusion and shortening of the cervical vertebrae. It is associated with shortness of neck, low hairline, and limited motion of head and neck.

2. Intervertebral disk herniation involves the prolapse of the nucleus pulposus through the defective annulus fibrosis into the vertebral canal. The nucleus pulposus impinges on spinal roots and results in root pain and radiculopathy.

3. Spina bifida occulta results from failure of the vertebral arches to form or fuse.

4. Spondylolisthesis occurs when the pedicles of the vertebral arches fail to fuse with the vertebral body. This allows the vertebral body to move anteriorly with respect to the vertebrae below it, causing **lordosis. Congenital spondylolisthesis** usually occurs at the L5-S1 vertebral level.

5. Hemivertebrae occur when wedges of vertebrae appear, usually situated laterally between two other vertebrae.

6. Vertebral bar occurs when there is a localized failure of segmentation on one side of the column, usually in a posterolateral site.

7. Block vertebra occurs when there is a lack of separation between two or more vertebrae, usually in the lumbar region.

8. Cleft vertebra occurs when a cleft develops in the vertebra, usually in a coronal or sagittal plane in the lumbar region.

9. Idiopathic scoliosis is a lateral deviation of the vertebral column that involves both deviation and rotation of vertebral bodies.

III Ribs

A. Development in general. Ribs develop from costal processes that form at all vertebral levels. However, only in the thoracic region do the costal processes grow into ribs.

B. Clinical correlations

1. Accessory lumbar ribs are the most common.

2. Accessory cervical ribs. These ribs are attached to the C7 vertebrae and may end either freely or attached to the thoracic cage. Accessory cervical ribs may put pressure on the lower trunk of the brachial plexus and subclavian artery, causing superior **thoracic outlet syndrome.**

IV # Sternum

A. **Development in general.** The sternum develops from two sternal bars that form in the ventral body wall independent of the ribs and clavicle. By week 8, the sternal bars fuse with each other in a craniocaudal direction to form the **manubrium, body,** and **xiphoid process.**

B. **Clinical correlations**
1. **Sternal cleft** occurs when the sternal bars do not fuse completely. It is fairly common and, if small, is generally of no clinical significance.
2. **Pectus excavatum (funnel chest)** is the most common chest anomaly, consisting of a depression of the chest wall that may extend from the manubrium to the xiphoid process. In addition to the typical cosmetic appearance, these individuals demonstrate cardiopulmonary restriction, drooped shoulders, protuberant abdomen, and scoliosis, such that early surgical intervention is generally recommended.

V # Bones of the Limbs and Limb Girdles

A. **Development in general.** The bones of the limbs and limb girdles develop from condensations of lateral plate mesoderm within the limb buds. The limb buds are visible at week 4 of development; the upper limb appears first. The limbs are well differentiated at week 8. The limb tip contains the **apical ectodermal ridge,** which exerts an inductive influence on limb growth and development.

B. **Clinical correlations**
1. **Polydactyly** is an autosomal dominant disorder characterized by the presence of extra digits on the hands and feet.
2. **Holt-Oram syndrome (heart-hand syndrome)** is an autosomal dominant disorder associated with chromosome 12 that causes anomalies of the upper limb and heart.
3. **Syndactyly** (webbed fingers or toes) is the most common limb anomaly and results from failure of the hand or foot webs to degenerate between the digits.
4. **Amelia** (an absence of one or two extremities) may result from the use, by the expectant mother, of the teratogen **thalidomide.**

VI # Osteogenesis. Osteogenesis occurs through the conversion of preexisting connective tissue (mesoderm) into bone. This process is called **ossification.** During development, two types of ossification occur:

A. **Intramembranous ossification** occurs in the embryo when mesoderm condenses into sheets of highly vascular connective tissue, which then **directly** form a primary ossification center. **Bones that form via intramembranous ossification are** the frontal bone, parietal bones, intraparietal part of occipital bone, maxilla, zygomatic bone, squamous part of temporal bone, palatine, vomer, and mandible.

B. **Endochondral ossification** occurs in the embryo when mesoderm first forms a hyaline cartilage model, which then develops a primary ossification center at the diaphysis. **Bones that form via endochondral ossification are** the ethmoid bone, sphenoid bone, petrous and mastoid parts of the temporal bone, basilar part of the occipital bone, incus, malleus, stapes, styloid process, hyoid bone, bones of the limbs, limb girdles, vertebrae, sternum, and ribs.

VII # General Skeletal Abnormalities (Figure 18-3)

A. **Achondroplasia (AC)** is the most prevalent form of dwarfism. AC is an autosomal dominant genetic disorder caused by a mutation in the gene for **fibroblast growth factor receptor 3 (FGFR3)** on chromosome 4p16. Pathological changes are observed at the epiphyseal

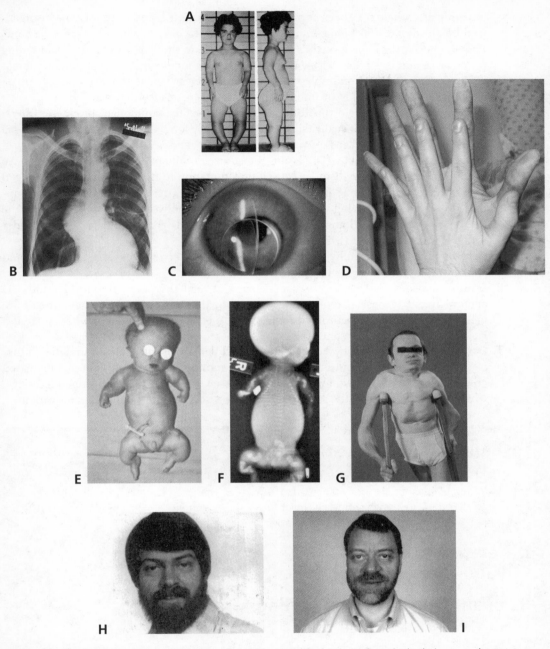

● **Figure 18.3 (A) Achondroplasia.** A 15-year-old girl with achondroplasia. Note the lordotic curve, short stature, short limbs and fingers, disproportionate trunk, bowed legs, relatively large head, prominent forehead, and deep nasal bridge. **(B–D) Marfan syndrome. (B)** AP radiograph shows hyperinflation, bullous changes, "tall" lungs, and a dilated, tortuous aorta. **(C)** Slit-lamp photomicrography shows ectopia lentis with microspherophakia. The lens is completely luxated into the anterior chamber of the eye, predisposing to pupillary block glaucoma. **(D)** Marfan syndrome is characterized by unusually tall stature, exceptionally long limbs, and arachnodactyly (elongated hands and feet with very slender digits). Note the exceptionally long and very slender fingers compared with those of a normal age-matched individual. **(E–G) Osteogenesis imperfecta. (E)** Infant with osteogenesis imperfecta. This newborn died immediately after birth from respiratory insufficiency. Note the lack of calcified calvaria, whereby the finger can easily indent the skull. Note the short, bowed upper and lower limbs. **(F)** Radiograph of an infant with osteogenesis imperfecta. Note the multiple bone fractures of the upper and lower limb, resulting in an accordion-like shortening of the limbs. **(G)** A man with osteogenesis imperfecta, showing the severe crippling deformities. **(H,I) Acromegaly. (H)** Photograph of a 22-year-old man before he developed telltale signs of acromegaly. **(I)** Photograph of the same man at age 39 with the distinct facial appearance of acromegaly.

growth plate, where the zones of proliferation and hypertrophy are narrow and disorganized. Horizontal struts of bone eventually grow into the growth plate and "seal" the bone, thereby preventing bone growth. These individuals are short in stature, with shortening of the arms and legs along with a disproportionately long trunk. Mental function is not affected. Chances of achondroplasia increase with increasing paternal age.

B. Marfan syndrome (MS) is an autosomal dominant genetic disorder caused by a mutation in the gene for the protein **fibrillin,** which is an essential component of **elastic fibers.** These individuals are unusually tall with exceptionally long, thin limbs; they have ectopia lentis (dislocation of the lens), severe nearsightedness, and heart valve incompetence.

C. Osteogenesis imperfecta (OI) is an autosomal dominant (types I–IV) or recessive (types II and III) genetic disorder caused by a mutation in the gene for **type I collagen** on chromosome 7q22 or 18q22. OI is characterized by extreme bone fragility with spontaneous fractures occurring when the fetus is still in the womb and blue sclerae of the eyes. Severe forms of OI are fatal in utero or during the early neonatal period. Milder forms of OI may be confused with child abuse.

D. Acromegaly results from hyperpituitarism. It is characterized by a large jaw, hands, and feet, and sometimes by gigantism.

E. Cretinism occurs when there is a deficiency in fetal thyroid hormone (T3 and T4) and/or thyroid agenesis. Cretinism results in growth retardation, skeletal abnormalities, mental retardation, and neurological disorders. It is rare except in areas where there is a lack of iodine in the water and soil.

F. Osteopetrosis is caused by markedly increased density of the skeleton due to a failure of osteoclastic activity and is associated with multiple fractures in spite of increased bone density. There are two forms of osteopetrosis: the first form is autosomal recessive, which is fatal in infancy; the second form is a less severe autosomal dominant variant.

Case Study 1

A frantic father rushes his 1-year-old daughter to your clinic saying that he thinks "my daughter's leg is broken." He says that "this is the third time that my daughter has broken a bone" and that his wife may be abusing the child while he is at work. The child's chart reveals that there were bone fractures at birth. What is the most likely diagnosis?

Differentials

- Child abuse, Marfan syndrome, osteogenesis imperfecta

Relevant Physical Exam Findings

- Short, deformed extremities
- Blue sclerae of the eyes
- Kyphoscoliosis

Relevant Lab Findings

- Multiple healed fractures on radiographs
- Deficiency of type I collagen

Diagnosis

- Osteogenesis imperfecta. The clinical finding of multiple occurrences of broken bones in an infant would immediately suggest some form of child abuse or osteogenesis imperfecta. In this case, child abuse would be ruled out due to the daughter's physical and lab findings.

Case Study 2

A 22-year-old man comes into the office complaining of blurred vision. He states that he has "not had problems seeing before" and remarks that "my dad and sister had the same problem around my age." What is the most likely diagnosis?

Differentials

- Infection, fatigue, Marfan syndrome

Relevant Physical Exam Findings

- Tall male with long, spidery fingers (arachnodactyly)
- Hyperextensive joints
- Arm span much greater than body height
- Dislocation of lens (ectopia lentis)

Relevant Lab Findings

- Chest CT shows dilated aortic root.
- Genetic testing reveals a mutation in fibrillin-1.

Diagnosis

- Marfan syndrome

Chapter 19

Muscular System

I Skeletal Muscle

A. Molecular events. Mesodermal (mesenchymal) cells within somites become committed to a muscle-forming cell line through a poorly understood mechanism to form **myogenic cells.** Myogenic cells enter the cell cycle (i.e., undergo mitosis), which is stimulated by **FGF** (fibroblast growth factor) and **TGF-β** (transforming growth factor beta). **Pax-3** and **myf-5** stimulate myogenic cells to begin expression of **MyoD** (a helix-loop-helix transcription factor). MyoD binds to the **E box** (CANNTG) on DNA, which removes the myogenic cells from the cell cycle (i.e., mitosis stops) and switches on **muscle-specific genes** to form **postmitotic myoblasts.** Myoblasts begin to synthesize **actin** and **myosin** while they fuse with each other to form multinucleated **myotubes.** Myotubes synthesize **actin, myosin, troponin, tropomyosin,** and **other muscle proteins.** These proteins aggregate into **myofibrils,** at which stage the cells are called **muscle fibers.** Since muscle fibers are postmitotic, further growth is accomplished by means of **satellite cells,** which operate by poorly understood mechanisms.

B. Paraxial mesoderm is a thick plate of mesoderm on each side of the midline. The paraxial mesoderm becomes organized into segments known as **somitomeres,** which form in a craniocaudal sequence. **Somitomeres 1–7** do not form somites but contribute mesoderm to the head and neck region (pharyngeal arches). **The remaining somitomeres** further condense in a craniocaudal sequence to form 42–44 pairs of somites of the trunk region. The somites closest to the caudal end eventually disappear to give a final count of approximately **35 pairs of somites.** Somites further differentiate into the sclerotome (cartilage and bone component), myotome (muscle component), and dermatome (dermis of skin component).

C. Head and neck musculature is derived from somitomeres 1–7 of the head and neck region, which participate in the formation of the pharyngeal arches.

   1. Extraocular muscles are derived from somitomeres 1, 2, 3, and 5. Somitomeres 1, 2, and 3 are called **preoptic myotomes.** The extraocular muscles are innervated by CN III, CN IV, and CN VI.

   2. Tongue muscles are derived from **occipital myotomes.** The tongue muscles are innervated by CN XII.

D. Trunk musculature (Figure 19-1) is derived from myotomes in the trunk region. Each myotome partitions into a dorsal **epimere** and a ventral **hypomere.**

   1. The epimere develops into the extensor muscles of the neck and vertebral column (e.g., erector spinae). The epimere is innervated by **dorsal rami of spinal nerves.**

   2. The hypomere develops into the scalene, prevertebral, geniohyoid, infrahyoid, intercostal, and abdominal muscles; the lateral and ventral flexors of the vertebral column; the quadratus lumborum; and the pelvic diaphragm. The hypomere is innervated by **ventral rami of spinal nerves.**

E. Limb musculature is derived from myotomes (somites) in the upper and lower limb bud regions. This mesoderm migrates into the limb bud and forms a **posterior condensation** and an **anterior condensation.**

   1. The posterior condensation develops into the **extensor and supinator musculature of the upper limb** and the **extensor and abductor musculature of the lower limb.**

   2. The anterior condensation develops into the **flexor and pronator musculature of the upper limb** and the **flexor and adductor musculature of the lower limb.**

II Smooth Muscle of the gastrointestinal tract and the tunica media of blood vessels is derived from mesoderm.

III Cardiac Muscle is derived from mesoderm that surrounds the primitive heart tube and becomes the myocardium.

IV Clinical Considerations (Figure 19-1)

A. Prune-belly syndrome occurs when the **abdominal musculature** is absent or very hypoplastic, most likely involving cells of the hypomere.

B. Poland syndrome is a relatively uncommon chest anomaly characterized by the **partial or complete absence of the pectoralis major muscle.** In addition, these individuals may demonstrate partial agenesis of the ribs and sternum, mammary gland aplasia, or absence of the latissimus dorsi and serratus anterior muscles.

C. Congenital torticollis (wryneck) occurs when the **sternocleidomastoid muscle** is abnormally shortened, causing rotation and tilting of the head. It may be caused by injury to the sternocleidomastoid muscle during childbirth, formation of a hematoma, and eventual fibrosis of the muscle.

D. Duchenne muscular dystrophy (DMD). DMD is an **X-linked recessive disorder** caused by a mutation in the gene for **dystrophin** on the short arm of chromosome X (Xp21). X-linked recessive inheritance means that males who inherit only one defective copy of the DMD gene from the mother have the disease. Dystrophin anchors the cytoskeleton (actin) of skeletal muscle cells to the extracellular matrix through a transmembrane protein (α-dystroglycan and β-dystroglycan) and stabilizes the cell membrane. A mutation of the DMD gene destroys the ability of dystrophin to anchor actin to the extracellular matrix. The characteristic dysfunction in DMD is **progressive muscle weakness and wasting.** Death occurs as a result of cardiac or respiratory failure, usually in the late teens or early twenties.

E. Becker muscular dystrophy is a less severe form of Duchenne muscular dystrophy.

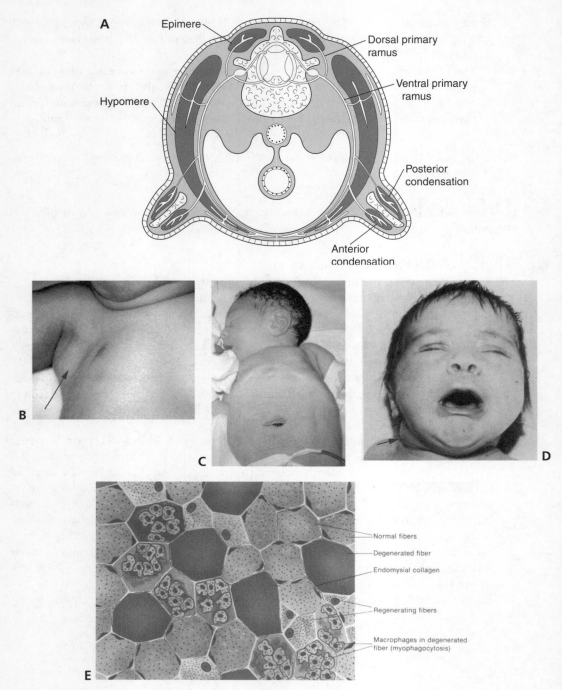

● **Figure 19.1 (A) Drawing of a transverse section through the thorax and limb bud, showing the muscles of the epimere, hypomere, and limb bud.** The limb bud musculature develops from mesoderm of various myotomes. The epimeric muscles are innervated by dorsal primary rami, and the hypomeric and limb muscles are innervated by ventral primary rami of spinal nerves. **(B) Prune-belly syndrome.** The absence of the abdominal musculature is apparent, causing a widening of the flanks. **(C) Poland syndrome.** The absence of the right pectoralis major muscle (arrow) and loss of the right anterior axillary fold is apparent. **(D) Congenital torticollis (wryneck).** A fibrous mass (arrow) in the right sternocleidomastoid muscle is apparent (arrow). **(E) Duchenne muscular dystrophy (DMD; Gomori trichrome stain).** Some muscle fibers are slightly larger and darker than normal, which represents overcontracted, normal myofibrillar segments situated between degenerated myofibrillar segments. Some muscle fibers are packed with macrophages (myophagocytosis) in the process of removing degenerated muscle cells. Some muscle fibers are smaller than normal, with large vesicular nuclei, prominent nucleoli, and a granular cytoplasm. These muscle fibers represent regenerating muscle fibers. The endomysium is thickened.

Case Study

A mother brings her 12-year-old son to the clinic because the child is feeling weakness in his legs. The mother says "he can't run as good as he used to." She also says it's gotten so bad that when "he's sitting down, he has to put his hands on his thighs to help himself stand up." What is the most likely diagnosis?

Differentials

- Glycogen storage disease, Duchenne muscular dystrophy, Becker muscular dystrophy

Relevant Physical Exam Findings

- Rapidly progressive muscle weakness with frequent falls
- Muscle wasting in the legs and pelvis, progressing to shoulders and neck
- Pseudohypertrophy of calf muscles

Relevant Lab Findings

- No sign of myoglobinuria
- Highly elevated CPK
- EMG (electromyography) showing weakness due to muscle tissue destruction and not nerve damage
- Confirmation of Duchenne muscular dystrophy by muscle biopsy
- Genetic mutation of the DMD gene located on the short arm (p) of chromosome X in band 21 (Xp21)

Diagnosis

- Duchenne muscular dystrophy. The description of how the boy arises from a seated position is called the Gower maneuver, which is classically seen in this condition. Becker muscular dystrophy normally begins around the third decade of life, whereas Duchenne can begin much earlier. McArdle disease would also be excluded because there was no sign of myoglobinuria, which would be a result of muscle glycogen phosphorylase deficiency.

Chapter 20

Pregnancy

I Endocrinology of Pregnancy

A. Human chorionic gonadotropin (hCG)

1. **Definition.** hCG is a glycoprotein hormone produced by the **syncytiotrophoblasts,** which stimulates the production of progesterone by the corpus luteum (i.e., maintains corpus luteum function). hCG can be assayed in **maternal blood at day 8** or **maternal urine at day 10** using a radioimmunoassay with antibodies directed against the β-subunit of hCG. This is the basis of the early-pregnancy test kits purchased over the counter.

2. **Quantitative hCG dating of pregnancy.** During weeks 1–6 of a normal pregnancy, hCG levels will increase by about 70% every 48 hours.

0–2 weeks:	0–250 mIU/mL
2–4 weeks:	100–5000 mIU/mL
1–2 months:	4000–200,000 mIU/mL
2–3 months:	8000–100,000 mIU/mL
2nd trimester:	4000–75,000 mIU/mL
3rd trimester:	1000–5000 mIU/mL

3. **Other tests using hCG.** Low hCG levels may predict a spontaneous abortion or indicate an ectopic pregnancy. Elevated hCG levels may indicate a multiple pregnancy, hydatidiform mole, or gestational trophoblastic neoplasia.

B. Human placental lactogen (hPL) is a protein hormone produced by the **placenta** that induces lipolysis, thereby elevating levels of free fatty acid in the mother. It is considered the "growth hormone" of the latter half of pregnancy. hPL can be assayed in **maternal blood at week 6.** hPL levels vary with placental mass (i.e., they may indicate a multiple pregnancy) and rapidly disappear from maternal blood after delivery.

C. Prolactin (PRL)—a protein hormone produced by the **maternal adenohypophysis, fetal adenohypophysis,** and **decidual tissue of the uterus**—prepares the mammary glands for lactation. PRL can be assayed in **maternal blood throughout pregnancy** or later in **amniotic fluid.** Near term, PRL levels rise to a maximum of about 100 ng/mL (normal nonpregnant PRL levels range between 8 and 25 ng/mL).

D. Progesterone (PG) is a steroid hormone produced by the **corpus luteum** until week 8 and then by the **placenta** until birth. PG does the following:

1. PG prepares the endometrium for implantation (nidation) and maintains the endometrium.

2. PG is used by the fetal adrenal cortex as a precursor for corticosteroid and mineralocorticoid synthesis.

3. PG is used by the fetal testes as a precursor for testosterone synthesis.

E. Estrone, estradiol, and estriol

1. Little is known about the specific function of these steroid hormones in the mother or fetus during pregnancy. These steroid hormones are produced by a complex series of steps involving the **maternal liver, placenta, fetal adrenal gland,** and **fetal liver,** as indicated below:

   a. Cholesterol from the maternal liver is converted to pregnenolone by the placenta.

   b. Pregnenolone is converted to pregnenolone sulfate.

   c. Pregnenolone sulfate is converted to dehydroepiandrosterone sulfate (DHEA-SO_4) by the fetal adrenal gland.

   d. DHEA-SO_4 is converted to estrone and estradiol by the placenta.

   e. DHEA-SO_4 is also converted to 16 α-hydroxy DHEA-SO_4 by the fetal liver.

   f. 16 α-hydroxy DHEA-SO_4 is converted to estriol by the placenta.

2. **Estrone** is a fairly weak estrogen.

3. **Estradiol** is the most potent estrogen.

4. **Estriol** is a very weak estrogen but is produced in very high amounts during pregnancy. Estriol can be assayed in **maternal blood** (shows a distinct diurnal variation with peak amounts early in the morning) and **maternal urine** (24-hour urine sample shows no diurnal variation). Significant amounts of estriol are produced at month 3 (i.e., early second trimester) and continue to rise until birth. Maternal urinary levels of estriol have long been recognized as a **reliable index of fetal-placental function,** since estriol production is dependent on a normal-functioning fetal adrenal cortex, fetal liver, and placenta.

II Pregnancy Dating.

The **estimated date of confinement (EDC)** is based on the assumption that a woman has a 28-day cycle with ovulation on day 14 or day 15. In general, the duration of a normal pregnancy is **280 days (40 weeks) from the first day of the last menstrual period (LMP).** A common method to determine the EDC (Naegele's rule) is to count back 3 months from the first day of the LMP and then add 1 year and 7 days; this method is reasonably accurate in women with regular menstrual cycles.

III Pregnancy Milestones

A. The **first trimester** extends from the last menstrual period through week 12. Important events that occur are as follows:

1. At days 8–10, a positive pregnancy test is obtained by hCG assay.

2. At week 12, the uterine fundus is palpable at the pubic symphysis; the Doppler fetal heart rate is first audible.

B. The **second trimester** extends from the end of the first trimester through week 27. Important events that occur are as follows:

1. At weeks 14–18, when suspicion of fetal chromosomal abnormalities exists, amniocentesis is performed.

2. At week 16, the uterine fundus is palpable midway between the pubic symphysis and umbilicus.

3. At weeks 16–18, the first fetal movements occur (**quickening**) in a woman's second or later pregnancy.

4. At weeks 17–20, the fetal heart rate is audible with a fetoscope.

5. At week 18, female and male external genitalia can be distinguished by ultrasound (i.e., sex determination).

6. At weeks 18–20, first fetal movements occur (**quickening**) in a woman's first pregnancy.

7. At week 20, the uterine fundus is palpable at the umbilicus.

8. At weeks 25–27, the lungs become capable of respiration; surfactant is produced by type II pneumocytes. There is a 70%–80% chance of survival for infants born at the end of the second trimester. If death occurs, it is generally as a result of lung immaturity and associated respiratory distress syndrome (hyaline membrane disease).

9. At week 27, the fetus weighs about 1000 grams (a little more than 2 pounds).

C. The **third trimester** extends from the end of the second trimester until term or week 40. Important events that occur are as follows:

1. The pupillary light reflex is present.
2. Descent of the fetal head to the pelvic inlet (called **lightening**) occurs.
3. Rupture of the amniochorionic membrane occurs, with labor usually beginning about 24 hours later.
4. The fetus weighs about 3300 grams (about 7–7.5 pounds).

IV **Prenatal Diagnostic Procedures.** Prenatal diagnosis is indicated in about **8%** of all pregnancies. Prenatal diagnostic procedures include:

A. **Ultrasonography.** Ultrasonography is commonly used to date a pregnancy, diagnose a multiple pregnancy, assess fetal growth, determine placental location, determine position and lie of the fetus, detect certain congenital anomalies, and monitor needle or catheter insertion during amniocentesis and chorionic villus biopsy. In obstetric ultrasonography, frequencies of 2.25–5.0 mHz are used for good tissue differentiation. The term **"anechoic"** refers to tissues with few or no echoes (e.g., bladder, brain, cavities, amniotic fluid). The term **"echogenic"** refers to tissues with a high capacity to reflect ultrasound. **B-scan ultrasonography** consists of an **A-mode** and **M-mode** (which provide precise measurements) and **time position scan** with a permanent record of cinephotography. **Real-time ultrasonography** provides an easy, immediate, and definitive demonstration of fetal life.

B. **Amniocentesis** is a transabdominal sampling of **amniotic fluid** and **fetal cells.** Amniocentesis is performed at weeks 14–18 and is indicated in the following situations: the woman is over 35 years of age, a previous child has a chromosomal anomaly, one parent is a known carrier of a translocation or inversion, one or both parents are known carriers of an X-linked recessive or autosomal recessive trait, or there is a history of neural tube defects. The sample obtained is used in the following studies:

1. **α-Fetoprotein assay,** used to diagnose neural tube defects.
2. **Spectrophotometric assay of bilirubin,** used to diagnose hemolytic disease of the newborn (i.e., erythroblastosis fetalis) due to Rh incompatibility.
3. **Lecithin-sphingomyelin (L/S) ratio and phosphatidylglycerol assay,** used to determine lung maturity of the fetus.
4. **DNA analysis.** A wide variety of DNA methodologies are available [e.g., karyotype analysis, Southern blotting, or RFLP analysis (restriction fragment length polymorphism)] to diagnose chromosomal abnormalities and single-gene defects.

C. **Chorionic villus biopsy** is a transabdominal or transcervical sampling of the chorionic villi to obtain a large amount of **fetal cells** for DNA analysis. Chorionic villus biopsy is performed at weeks 6–11 (i.e., much earlier than amniocentesis), thereby providing an early source of fetal cells for DNA analysis.

D. **Percutaneous umbilical blood sampling (PUBS)** is a sampling of **fetal blood** from the umbilical cord.

V **Fetal Distress During Labor (Intrapartum)** is defined in terms of **fetal hypoxia** and measured by changes in either **fetal heart rate (FHR)** or **fetal scalp capillary pH.** The normal baseline FHR is 120–160 beats per minute. However, fetal hypoxia causes a decrease in FHR (or **fetal bradycardia**)—that is, an **FHR less than 120 beats per minute.** The normal fetal scalp capillary pH is 7.25–7.35. However, fetal hypoxia causes a decrease in pH— that is, a **pH below 7.20.**

TABLE 20-1	ASSESSING THE APGAR SCORE			
Characteristic	0	1	2	Example[a]
Appearance, color	Blue, pale	Body pink, extremities blue	Completely pink	1
Pulse, heart rate	Absent	<100 bpm	>100 bpm	2
Grimace reflex, irritability	No response	Grimace	Vigorous crying	0
Activity, muscle tone	Flaccid	Some flexion of extremities	Active motion, flexed extremities	0
Respiratory effort	None	Weak, irregular	Good, crying	1
Apgar score				4

[a]Clinical example: A newborn infant at 5 minutes after birth has a pink body but blue extremities (score 1); a heart rate of 125 bpm (score 2); shows no grimace or reflex (score 0); has flaccid muscle tone (score 0); has weak, irregular breathing (score 1). The total Apgar score is 4. This infant needs ventilation and temperature support.

VI. The Apgar Score.
Table 20-1 assesses five characteristics (**a**ppearance, **p**ulse, **g**rimace, **a**ctivity, **r**espiratory effort) in the newborn infant in order to determine which infants need resuscitation.

The Apgar score is calculated at 1 min and 5 min after birth. To obtain an Apgar score, score 0, 1, or 2 for the five characteristics and add them together.

A. An **Apgar score of 0–3** indicates a life-threatening situation.
B. An **Apgar score of 4–6** indicates that temperature and ventilation support is needed.
C. An **Apgar score of 7–10** indicates a normal situation.

VII. The Puerperium
extends from immediately after delivery of the baby until the reproductive tract returns to the nonpregnant state in approximately 4–6 weeks. Important events that occur are:

A. Involution of the uterus.
B. Afterpains due to uterine contractions.
C. Uterine discharge (lochia).
D. In nonlactating women, menstrual flow returns within 6–8 weeks postpartum and ovulation returns 2–4 weeks postpartum.
E. In lactating women, ovulation may return within 10 weeks postpartum. Birth control protection afforded by lactation is assured for only 6 weeks, after which time pregnancy is possible.

VIII. Lactation
A. **During pregnancy,** hPL, PRL, progesterone, estrogens, cortisol, and insulin stimulate the growth of **lactiferous ducts** and the proliferation of epithelial cells to form **alveoli;** alveoli secrete **colostrum.**
B. **After delivery of the baby,** lactation is initiated by a decrease in progesterone and estrogens along with the release of PRL from the adenohypophysis. This initiates **milk production.**
C. **During suckling,** a stimulus from the breast inhibits the release of PRL-inhibiting factor from the hypothalamus, thereby causing a **surge in PRL,** which increases milk production. In addition, stimulation of the nipples during suckling causes a **surge of oxytocin,** which causes the expulsion of accumulated milk ("milk letdown") by stimulating myoepithelial cells.

Chapter 21

Numerical Chromosomal Anomalies

I **Polyploidy** is the addition of an extra haploid set or sets of chromosomes (i.e., 23) to the normal diploid set of chromosomes (i.e., 46).

A. **Triploidy** is a condition whereby cells contain **69 chromosomes.** It results in spontaneous abortion of the conceptus or brief survival of the live-born infant after birth. Triploidy occurs as a result of either a **failure of meiosis in a germ cell** (e.g., fertilization of a diploid egg by a haploid sperm) or **dispermy** (two sperm that fertilize one egg).

B. **Tetraploidy is** a condition whereby cells contain **92 chromosomes.** It results in spontaneous abortion of the conceptus. Tetraploidy occurs as a result of **failure of the first cleavage division.**

II **Aneuploidy** **(Figure 21-1)** is the addition of one chromosome (**trisomy**) or loss of one chromosome (**monosomy**). Trisomy results in spontaneous abortion of the conceptus. However, trisomy 13 (Patau syndrome), trisomy 18 (Edwards syndrome), trisomy 21 (Down syndrome), and Klinefelter syndrome (47, XXY) are found in the live-born population. Monosomy results in spontaneous abortion of the conceptus. However, monosomy X chromosome (45, X; Turner syndrome) is found in the live born population. Aneuploidy occurs as a result of **nondisjunction during meiosis.**

A. **Trisomy 13 (Patau syndrome)** is characterized by profound mental retardation, congenital heart defects, cleft lip and palate, omphalocele, and polydactyly. These infants usually die soon after birth.

B. **Trisomy 18 (Edwards syndrome)** is characterized by mental retardation, congenital heart defects, small facies and prominent occiput, overlapping fingers, and rocker-bottom heels. These infants usually die soon after birth.

C. **Trisomy 21 (Down syndrome)** is characterized by moderate mental retardation (it is the leading cause of inherited mental retardation), microcephaly, microphthalmia, colobomata, cataracts and glaucoma, flat nasal bridge, epicanthic folds, protruding tongue, simian crease in hand, increased nuchal skin folds, appearance of an "X" across the face when the baby cries because the upward-slanting palpebral fissures run in a line with the nasolabial folds, and congenital heart defects. Alzheimer neurofibrillary tangles and plaques are found in Down syndrome patients after 30 years of age. Acute megakaryocytic leukemia (AMKL) is frequently present.

1. Trisomy 21 is the most common type of trisomy, whose frequency increases with **advanced maternal age.**

2. Trisomy 21 is associated with **low α-fetoprotein levels** in amniotic fluid or maternal serum.

3. A specific region on chromosome 21—called **DSCR (Down syndrome critical region)**—seems to be markedly associated with numerous features of trisomy 21. The following genes have been mapped to the DSCR (although their role is far from clear): carbonyl reductase, SIM2 (a transcription factor), p60 subunit of chromatin

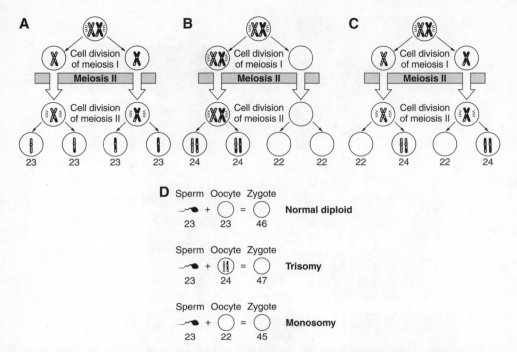

D Sperm Oocyte Zygote

Normal diploid
23   23   46

Trisomy
23   24   47

Monosomy
23   22   45

● **Figure 21.1 (A) Normal meiotic divisions (I and II) producing gametes with 23 chromosomes. (B) Nondisjunction occurring in meiosis I, producing gametes with 24 and 22 chromosomes. (C) Nondisjunction occurring in meiosis II, producing gametes with 24 and 22 chromosomes. (D) Although nondisjunction may occur in either spermatogenesis or oogenesis, there is a higher frequency of nondisjunction in oogenesis.** In this schematic, nondisjunction in oogenesis in depicted. If an abnormal oocyte (24 chromosomes) is fertilized by a normal sperm (23 chromosomes), a zygote with 47 chromosomes is produced (i.e., trisomy). If an abnormal oocyte (22 chromosomes) is fertilized by a normal sperm (23 chromosomes), a zygote with 45 chromosomes is produced (i.e., monosomy).

assembly factor, holocarboxylase synthetase, ERG (a proto-oncogene), GIRK2 (a K$^+$ ion channel), and PEP19 (a Ca^{2+}-dependent signal transducer).

4. Trisomy 21 may also be caused by a chromosomal translocation between chromosomes 14 and 21 [i.e., t(14;21)].

D. **Klinefelter syndrome (47, XXY)** is a trisomic condition **found only in males** and characterized by varicose veins, arterial and venous leg ulcers, scant body and pubic hair, male hypogonadism, sterility with fibrosis of seminiferous tubules, marked decrease in testosterone levels, elevated gonadotropin levels, gynecomastia, dull mentality, antisocial behavior, delayed speech as a child, and eunuchoid habitus.

E. **Turner syndrome (monosomy X; 45, X)** is a monosomic condition **found only in females** and characterized by short stature, low-set ears, ocular hypertelorism, ptosis, low posterior hairline, webbed neck due to a remnant of a fetal cystic hygroma, congenital hypoplasia of lymphatics causing peripheral edema of hands and feet, shield chest, pinpoint nipples, congenital heart defects, aortic coarctation, female hypogonadism, and ovarian fibrous streaks (i.e., infertility). This syndrome is a common cause of primary amenorrhea.

III ## Selected Photographs

A. Trisomy 13 (Patau syndrome; Figure 21-2A,B)
B. Trisomy 18 (Edwards syndrome; Figure 21-2C,D)
C. Trisomy 21 (Down syndrome; Figure 21-2E–G)
D. Klinefelter syndrome (Figure 21-2H)
E. Turner syndrome (Figure 21-2I,J)

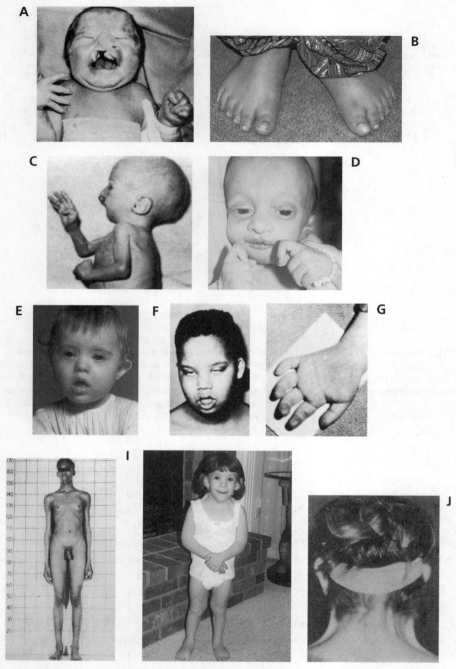

● **Figure 21.2 (A,B) Trisomy 13 (Patau syndrome).** The key features of trisomy 13 are microcephaly with sloping forehead, scalp defects, microphthalmia, cleft lip and palate, polydactyly, fingers flexed and overlapping, and cardiac malformations. **(C,D) Trisomy 18 (Edwards syndrome).** The key features of trisomy 18 are low birth weight, lack of subcutaneous fat, prominent occiput, narrow forehead, small palpebral fissures, low-set and malformed ears, micrognathia, short sternum, and cardiac malformations. **(E–G) Trisomy 21 (Down syndrome). (E,F)** Photographs of a young child and boy with Down syndrome. Note the flat nasal bridge, prominent epicanthic folds, oblique palpebral fissures, low-set and shell-like ears, and protruding tongue. Other associated features include generalized hypotonia, transverse palmar creases (simian lines), shortening and incurving of the fifth fingers (clinodactyly), Brushfield spots, and mental retardation. **(G)** Photograph of a hand in Down syndrome showing the simian crease. **(H) Klinefelter syndrome (47, XXY).** Photograph of a young man with Klinefelter syndrome. Note the hypogonadism, eunuchoid habitus, and gynecomastia. **(I,J) Turner syndrome (45, X).** Photograph of a 3-year-old girl with Turner syndrome. Note the webbed neck due to delayed maturation of lymphatics, short stature, and broad shield chest.

Case Study

A woman comes in with her 16-year-old daughter. The daughter states that she has "not had a menstrual period yet," is not sexually active, and is not on any form of birth control. What is the most likely diagnosis?

Differentials

- Congenital adrenal hyperplasia, Turner syndrome, pituitary tumor, pituitary insufficiency

Relevant Physical Exam Findings

- Female with short stature
- Webbed neck
- Absent menstruation (primary amenorrhea)
- Shield-shaped chest

Relevant Lab Findings

- Karyotyping showing 45, XO
- Ultrasound showing small or underdeveloped female reproductive organs
- CT head scan revealing no sign of tumor

Diagnosis

- Turner syndrome. A webbed neck, shield-shaped chest, and 45, XO karyotype are classic signs of Turner syndrome.

Chapter 22

Structural Chromosomal Anomalies

I   Deletions are losses of chromatin from a chromosome. The following are clinical examples caused by deletions.

- **A. Chromosome 4p deletion (Wolf-Hirschhorn syndrome)** is caused by a deletion in the short arm of **chromosome 4 (4p16).** This deletion is characterized by prominent forehead and broad nasal root ("Greek warrior helmet"), short philtrum, downturned mouth, congenital heart defects, growth retardation, and severe mental retardation.
- **B. Chromosome 5p deletion (cri-du-chat or cat-cry syndrome)** is caused by a deletion in the short arm of **chromosome 5 (5p15).** This deletion is characterized by a round facies, a cat-like cry, congenital heart defects (e.g., VSDs), microcephaly, and mental retardation.
- **C. Ring chromosome 14** is caused when **chromosome 14** forms a ring structure with breakpoints at **14p11** and **14q32.** This deletion is characterized by mild dysmorphic features, frequent seizures, and variable mental retardation.

II   Microdeletions are losses of chromatin from a chromosome that can be detected only by high-resolution banding. The following are clinical examples caused by microdeletions.

- **A. Prader-Willi syndrome (PW)** is caused by a microdeletion in the long arm of **chromosome 15 (15q11-13),** derived from the **father.** PW is characterized by hyperphagia (insatiable appetite), hypogonadism, hypotonia, obesity, short stature, small hands and feet, behavior problems (rage, violence), and mild-to-moderate mental retardation. PW illustrates the phenomenon of **genomic imprinting,** which is the differential expression of genes depending on the parent of origin. Clearly, both paternal and maternal genes are necessary and complementary for normal development to occur. This is consistent with the view that some genes are differentially activated or inactivated (i.e., imprinted) during gametogenesis. The mechanism of inactivation (or genomic imprinting) involves **DNA methylation of cytosine nucleotides** during gametogenesis resulting in transcriptional inactivation. Other examples that highlight the role of genomic imprinting include **hydatidiform moles** and **Beckwith-Wiedemann syndrome.** The counterpart of PW is **Angelman syndrome.**
- **B. Angelman syndrome (AS; "happy puppet" syndrome)** is caused by a microdeletion in the long arm of **chromosome 15 (15q11-13),** derived from the **mother.** AS is characterized by gait ataxia (stiff, jerky, unsteady, upheld arms), seizures, a happy disposition with inappropriate laughter, and severe mental retardation (only 5- to 10-word vocabulary). AS is an example of **genomic imprinting** (see above). The counterpart of AS is **Prader-Willi syndrome.**
- **C. DiGeorge syndrome (DS)** is caused by a microdeletion in the long arm of **chromosome 22 (22q11),** which is also called the **DiGeorge chromosomal region (DGCR).** DS occurs when **pharyngeal pouches 3 and 4** fail to differentiate into the thymus and

parathyroid glands. DS is usually accompanied by facial anomalies resembling first arch syndrome (micrognathia, low-set ears) due to abnormal migration of neural crest cells, cardiovascular anomalies due to abnormal migration of neural crest cells during formation of the aorticopulmonary septum, immunodeficiency due to absence of the thymus gland, and hypocalcemia due to absence of the parathyroid glands. DS has a phenotypic and genotypic similarity to **velocardiofacial syndrome (VCFS);** that is, both DS and VCFS are manifestations of a microdeletion at 22q11. The following genes have been mapped to 22q11 or the DGCR (although their role is far from clear): catechol-O-methyltransferase (COMT, an enzyme used in catecholamine metabolism), GpIbb (the receptor for von Willebrand factor), DGCR3 (a leucine zipper transcription factor), and citrate transport protein (CTP).

D. **Miller-Dieker syndrome (MD, agyria, lissencephaly)** is caused by a microdeletion in the short arm of **chromosome 17p13.3.** MD is characterized by lissencephaly (smooth brain—i.e., no gyri), microcephaly, and a high furrowing forehead; death occurs early. Lissencephaly should not be mistakenly diagnosed in the case of premature infants whose brains have not yet developed an adult pattern of gyri (gyri begin to appear normally at about week 28).

E. **WAGR syndrome** is caused by a microdeletion in the short arm of **chromosome 11p13,** where the **WT1 gene** (Wilms tumor gene 1) is located. WT1 encodes for a zinc-finger DNA-binding protein that is required for normal embryological development of the genitourinary system. WT1 isoforms synergize with **SF-1** (steroidogenic factor-1), a nuclear receptor that regulates the transcription of a number of genes involved in reproduction, steroidogenesis, and male sexual development. WAGR is characterized by: **W**ilms tumor, **a**niridia (absence of the iris), **g**enitourinary abnormalities (e.g., gonadoblastoma), and mental **r**etardation. Since the WAGR syndrome involves the deletion of a series of adjacent genes, it is a good example of a **contiguous gene syndrome.**

F. **Williams syndrome (WS)** is caused by a microdeletion in the long arm of **chromosome 7q11.23,** where the **ELN gene (elastin gene)** and **LIMK1 gene** are located. The ELN gene encodes for elastin protein, which is an important component of elastic fibers of connective tissue. The LIMK1 gene encodes for a brain-expressed kinase that seems to be involved in visual-spatial cognition. WS is characterized by facial dysmorphology (e.g., prominent lips, wide mouth, periorbital fullness of subcutaneous tissues, short palpebral fissures, short upturned nose, long philtrum), congenital heart defects (e.g., supravalvular aortic stenosis, pulmonic valvular stenosis, septal defects), renal abnormalities, hoarse voice, and mild mental deficiency with uneven cognitive disabilities.

III **Translocations** result from breakage and exchange of segments between chromosomes. The following are clinical examples caused by translocations.

A. **Robertsonian translocation t(13q14q)** is caused by a translocation between the long arms (q) of chromosomes 13 and 14, where the breakpoint is near the centromere. The short arms (p) of chromosomes 13 and 14 are generally lost. Carriers of this Robertsonian translocation are **clinically normal,** since 13p and 14p, which are lost, contain only inert DNA and some rRNA (ribosomal RNA) genes, which occur in multiple copies on other chromosomes. This is the **most common translocation found in humans.**

B. **Robertsonian translocation t(14q21q)** is caused by a translocation between the long arms (q) of chromosomes 14 and 21, where the breakpoint is near the centromere; the short arms (p) of chromosomes 14 and 21 are generally lost. Carriers of this Robertsonian translocation are **clinically normal.** The clinical issue in this Robertsonian translocation occurs when the carriers produce gametes by meiosis and reproduce. Depending on how the chromosomes segregate during meiosis, conception can produce offspring with trisomy 21 (live birth), trisomy 14 (early miscarriage), monosomy 14 or 21 (early miscarriage), normal chromosome complement (live birth), or a t(14q21q) carrier (live birth). Consequently, a couple where one member is a t(14q21q) carrier may have a baby with trisomy 21 (Down syndrome) or recurrent miscarriages.

C. **Acute promyelocytic leukemia t(15;17)(q21;q21)** is caused by a reciprocal translocation between band q21 on chromosome 15 and band q21 on chromosome 17. This results in a fusion of the **promyelocyte gene (PML gene)** on chromosome 15q21 with the **retinoic acid receptor gene (RARα gene)** on chromosome 17q21, thereby forming the *pml/rarα* **oncogene.** The **PML/RARα oncoprotein** (a transcription factor) blocks the differentiation of promyelocytes to mature granulocytes such that there is continued proliferation of promyelocytes. This leukemia is characterized by coagulopathy and severe bleeding.

D. **Chronic myeloid leukemia t(9;22)(q34;q11)** is caused by a reciprocal translocation between band q34 on chromosome 9 and band q11 on chromosome 22. This is referred to as the **Philadelphia chromosome.** It results in a fusion of the **ABL gene** on chromosome 9q34 with the **BCR gene** on chromosome 22q11, thereby forming the *abl/bcr* **oncogene.** The **ABL/BCR oncoprotein** (a tyrosine kinase) has enhanced tyrosine kinase activity, which transforms hematopoietic precursor cells. This leukemia is characterized by an increased number of granulocytes in all stages of maturation and many mature neutrophils.

IV ## Unstable Expanding Repeat Mutations (Dynamic Mutations) Dynamic mutations are mutations that involve the **insertion of a repeat sequence** either outside or inside the gene. Dynamic mutations demonstrate a **threshold length. Below a certain threshold length,** the repeat sequence is stable, does not cause disease, and is propagated to successive generations without change in length. **Above a certain threshold length,** the repeat sequence is unstable, causes disease, and is propagated to successive generations in expanding lengths. The exact mechanism by which expansion of the repeat sequences occurs is not known. One of the hallmarks of diseases caused by these mutations is **anticipation,** which means the age of onset is lower and the degree of severity is worsened in successive generations. Dynamic mutations are divided into two categories:

A. **Highly expanded repeats outside the gene.** In this category of dynamic mutation, various repeat sequences (e.g., CGG, CCG, GAA, CTG, CCTG, ATTCT, or CCCCGCC-CCGCG) undergo very large expansions. Below threshold length expansions are ~ 5–50 repeats. Above threshold length expansions are ~100–1000 repeats. This category of dynamic mutations is characterized by the following clinical conditions.

1. **Fragile X syndrome (Martin-Bell syndrome).** Fragile X syndrome involves two mutation sites. Fragile X site A involves a 200–1000+ unstable repeat sequence of $(CGG)_n$ located in a 5' UTR of the FMR1 gene (fragile X mental retardation 1 gene) on chromosome Xq27.3. Fragile X site B involves a 200+ unstable repeat sequence of $(CCG)_n$ located in a promoter region of the FMR 1 gene on chromosome Xq28. **Fragile X syndrome** is an X-linked recessive genetic disorder caused by a fragile site on chromosome Xq27 or Xq28. The fragile site is observed when cells are cultured in a **folate-depleted** medium. The fragile site is produced by a CGG repeat mutation near the **FMR1 gene.** The FMR1 gene encodes for a protein called **FMRP** whose exact function is not known but has RNA-binding capability. Fragile X syndrome is the second leading cause of inherited mental retardation (Down syndrome is the number one cause). Fragile X syndrome is characterized by: mental

retardation (most severe in males), macroorchidism, speech delay, behavioral problems (e.g., hyperactivity, attention deficit), prominent jaw, and large, dysmorphic ears.

2. **Friedreich ataxia (FA).** FA involves a 200–1700 unstable repeat sequence of $(GAA)_n$ located in intron 1 of the frataxin gene on chromosome 9q13-a21.1. FA is an autosomal recessive genetic disorder caused by the unstable repeat sequence on chromosome 9q13-a21.1. The frataxin gene encodes for a protein called **frataxin,** a mitochondrial protein whose precise function is unknown but which appears to play a role in antioxidation. A longstanding hypothesis is that FA is a result of mitochondrial accumulation of iron, which may promote oxidative stress injury. FA is characterized by: degeneration of the posterior columns and spinocerebellar tracts, loss of sensory neurons in the dorsal root ganglion, ataxia of all four limbs, optic atrophy, swallowing dysfunction, pyramidal tract disease, cardiomyopathy (arrhythmias), and diabetes.

3. **Myotonic dystrophy (DM).** DM involves two mutation sites.
   a. **DM1** involves a 50–4000 unstable repeat sequence of $(CTG)_n$ located in a 3'UTR of the DM1 gene on chromosome 19q13. Myotonic dystrophy type 1 (DM1) is an autosomal dominant genetic disorder caused by the unstable repeat sequence on chromosome 19q13. The DM1 gene encodes for a **serine threonine protein kinase.** DM1 is characterized by: myotonia (delayed muscle relaxation after contraction), cataracts, cardiomyopathy with conduction defects, multiple endocrinopathies, and low intelligence or dementia.
   b. **DM2** involves a 75–11,000 unstable repeat sequence of $(CCTG)_n$ located in intron 1 of the DM2 gene on chromosome 3q21. Myotonic dystrophy type 2 (DM2 or proximal myotonic myopathy) is an autosomal dominant genetic disorder caused by the unstable repeat sequence on chromosome 3q21. The DM2 gene encodes for **zinc finger protein 9.** DM2 is characterized by: myalgia and painful muscle cramps, fluctuating weakness and stiffness, calf pseudohypertrophy, diabetes, hypothyroidism, cardiac conduction defects, deafness, and gastrointestinal symptoms.

4. **Spinocerebellar ataxia (SCA).** Numerous classification systems have been proposed for the autosomal dominant ataxias. Using a system based on genetic loci, numerous SCAs have been classified (SCA1-26; numbers continue to grow). SCA involves multiple mutation sites.
   a. **SCA8** involves a 110–500+ unstable repeat sequence of $(CTG)_n$ located in an RNA-coding gene (antisense RNA) on chromosome 13q21. SCA8 is an autosomal dominant genetic disorder caused by the unstable repeat sequence on chromosome 13q21. The SCA8 gene probably encodes for an **antisense RNA** that regulates a brain-specific actin-binding protein. SCA8 is characterized by: slow, progressive cerebellar ataxia affecting gait, speech, swallowing, limb movements, and eye movements; and cerebral atrophy.
   b. **SCA11** involves a 1000+ unstable repeat sequence of $(ATTCT)_n$ located in an intron sequence of the SCA11 gene on chromosome 15q14-q21. SCA11 is an autosomal dominant genetic disorder caused by the unstable repeat sequence on chromosome 15q13-q21. The SCA11 gene encodes for an **unknown protein or RNA.** SCA11 is characterized by: a relatively mild, pure cerebellar ataxia.

5. **Juvenile myoclonic epilepsy (JME).** JME involves a 40–80 unstable repeat sequence of $(CCCCGCCCCGCG)_n$ located in a promoter region of the GABRA 1 gene (α1 subunit of the gamma-aminobutyric acid receptor subtype A) on chromosome 21q22.3. JME is an autosomal recessive genetic disorder caused by the unstable repeat sequence

on chromosome 21q22.3. The GABRA 1 gene encodes for the **α1 subunit of the gamma-aminobutyric acid receptor subtype A.** JME is characterized by: myoclonic jerks (often upon awakening in the morning), absence seizures, and generalized tonic-clonic seizures typically seen in a healthy young teenager.

B. **Moderately expanded CAG repeats with the gene.** In this category of dynamic mutation, a CAG repeat sequence undergoes moderate expansions. Below threshold length expansions are ~10–30 repeats. Above threshold length expansions are ~40–200 repeats. Since CAG codes for the amino acid **glutamine,** a long tract of glutamines (polyglutamine tract) will be inserted into the amino acid sequence of the protein and causes the protein to aggregate within certain cells. This category of dynamic mutations is characterized by the following clinical conditions.

1. **Huntington disease (HD).** HD involves a 26-100+ unstable repeat sequence of $(CAG)_n$ located in an exon (or coding) sequence of the HD gene on chromosome 4p16.3. HD is an autosomal dominant genetic disorder caused by the CAG repeat sequence on chromosome 4p16.3. The HD gene encodes for a protein called **huntingtin,** a cytoplasmic protein present in neurons within the striatum, cerebral cortex, and cerebellum although its precise function is unknown. A primary manifestation is movement jerkiness most apparent at movement termination. HD is also characterized by: chorea, memory deficits, affective disturbances, personality changes, diffuse and marked atrophy (neuronal loss) of the neostriatum, and neuronal intranuclear aggregates.

2. **Kennedy syndrome (KS; spinobulbar muscular atrophy).** KS involves a 38–62 unstable repeat sequence of $(CAG)_n$ located in an exon (or coding) sequence of the AR gene (androgen receptor gene) on chromosome Xq21. KS is an X-linked recessive genetic disorder caused by the CAG repeat sequence on chromosome Xq21. The KS gene encodes for the **androgen receptor protein,** which is a member of the steroid-thyroid-retinoid superfamily of nuclear receptors. The CAG repeat mutation in the AR gene seems to be a gain of function mutation; there is a well-known syndrome called complete androgen insensitivity that is caused by a loss of function mutation in the AR gene. KS is characterized by: progressive loss of anterior motor neurons, late onset gynecomastia, defective spermatogenesis, and a hormonal profile consistent with androgen resistance. How this CAG repeat mutation causes the neurological deficits is unknown.

3. **Spinocerebellar ataxia (SCA).** Numerous classification systems have been proposed for the autosomal dominant ataxias. Using a system based on genetic loci, numerous SCAs have been classified (SCA1–26; numbers continue to grow). SCA involves multiple mutation sites.

a. **SCA1** involves a 39–83 unstable repeat sequence of $(CAG)_n$ located in an exon (or coding) sequence of the SCA1 gene on chromosome 6p23. SCA1 is an autosomal dominant genetic disorder caused by the CAG repeat sequence on chromosome 6p23. The SCA1 gene encodes for **ataxin-1,** whose function is not known. Ataxin-1 is phosphorylated on serine 776 by Akt kinase and this serine is crucial in mediating the pathogenesis of SCA1. SCA1 is characterized by: progressive cerebellar ataxia, dysarthria, bulbar dysfunction, and intranuclear aggregates.

b. **SCA2** involves a 32–77 unstable repeat sequence of $(CAG)_n$ located in an exon (or coding) sequence of the SCA2 gene on chromosome 12q24. SCA2 is an autosomal dominant genetic disorder caused by the CAG repeat sequence on chromosome 12q24. The SCA2 gene encodes for **ataxin-2,** which functions in RNA splicing. SCA2 is characterized by: progressive cerebellar ataxia, dysarthria, bulbar dysfunction, slow saccadic eye movements, and intracytoplasmic aggregates.

c. **SCA3 (Machado-Joseph disease; MJD)** involves a 62–86 unstable repeat sequence of $(CAG)_n$ located in an exon (or coding) sequence of the SCA3/MJD gene on chromosome 14q32.1. SCA3 is an autosomal dominant genetic disorder caused by the CAG repeat sequence on chromosome 14q32.1. The SCA3/MJD gene encodes for **ataxin-3,** whose function is unknown. SCA3 is characterized by: progressive cerebellar ataxia, dysarthria, bulbar dysfunction, extrapyramidal features including rigidity and dystonia, upper and lower motor neuron signs, cognitive impairments, and intranuclear aggregates.

d. **SCA6** involves a 21–30 unstable repeat sequence of $(CAG)_n$ located in an exon (or coding) sequence of the SCA6 gene on chromosome 19p13. SCA6 is an autosomal dominant genetic disorder caused by the CAG repeat sequence on chromosome 19q13. The SCA6 gene encodes for the **a-1A subunit of P/Q type calcium channel protein.** SCA6 is characterized by: progressive cerebellar ataxia, cerebellar atrophy, horizontal and vertical nystagmus, abnormal vestibuloocular reflex, and intracytoplasmic aggregates.

e. **SCA7** involves a 37–200 unstable repeat sequence of $(CAG)_n$ located in an exon (or coding) sequence of the SCA7 gene on chromosome 3p12-p21.1. SCA7 is an autosomal dominant genetic disorder caused by the CAG repeat sequence on chromosome 3p12-p21.1. The SCA7 gene encodes for **ataxin-7,** whose function is unknown. SCA7 is characterized by: progressive cerebellar ataxia, seizures, myoclonus, cardiac involvement, and vision loss.

f. **SCA17** involves a 47–63 unstable repeat sequence of $(CAG)_n$ located in an exon (or coding) sequence on the TBP gene (TATA-binding protein gene) on chromosome 6q27. SCA17 is an autosomal dominant genetic disorder caused by the CAG repeat sequence on chromosome 6q27. The SCA 17 gene encodes for **TATA-binding protein,** which is a general transcription factor. SCA17 is characterized by: progressive cerebellar ataxia and dementia, eventually leading to bradykinesia, dysmetria, dysdiadochokinesis, hyperreflexia, and paucity of movement.

C. **Trinucleotide repeat expansions.** In addition to the above mentioned dynamic mutations, there is another category of mutation that involves short, stable trinucleotide repeat expansions (not considered a dynamic mutation). This category of mutation is characterized by the following clinical conditions:

a. **Oropharyngeal muscular dystrophy (PABP2 gene)**
b. **Pseudoachondroplasia (COMP gene)**
c. **Synpolydactyly (HOXD 13 gene)**

V **Isochromosomes** occur when the centromere divides transversely (instead of longitudinally) such that one of the chromosome arms is duplicated and the other is lost. **Isochromosome Xq** is a clinical example caused by an isochromosome.

A. **Isochromosome Xq** is caused by a duplication of the long arm (q) and loss of the short arm (p) of chromosome X. This isochromosome is found in 20% of females with **Turner syndrome.** The occurrence of isochromosomes within any of the autosomes is generally a lethal situation.

VI **Inversions** are the reversal of the order of DNA between two breaks in chromosomes. **Pericentric inversions** occur on both sides of the centromere. **Paracentric inversions** occur on the same side of the centromere. Carriers of inversions are normal. The diagnosis of an inversion is generally a coincidental finding during prenatal testing or the repeated occurrence of spontaneous abortions or stillbirths.

Breakages are breaks in chromosomes due to sunlight (or UV) irradiation, ionizing irradiation, DNA cross-linking agents, or DNA damaging agents. These insults may cause **depurination of DNA, deamination of cytosine to uracil,** or **pyrimidine dimerization,** which must be repaired by DNA repair enzymes. The clinical importance of DNA repair enzymes is illustrated by some rare inherited diseases that involve genetic defects in DNA repair enzymes, such as the following.

A. **Xeroderma pigmentosum (XP)** is an autosomal recessive genetic disorder in which the affected individuals are hypersensitive to **sunlight (UV radiation).** XP is characterized by acute sun sensitivity with sunburn-like reaction, severe skin lesions around the eyes and eyelids, and malignant skin cancers (basal and squamous cell carcinomas and melanomas); most individuals so affected die by 30 years of age. XP is caused by the inability to remove pyrimidine dimers due to a genetic defect in one or more of the **nucleotide excision repair enzymes.** There are seven complementation groups in XP **(XPA-XPG).** The seven genes involved in the cause of XP include the **XPA gene,** located on chromosome 9q22.3, which encodes for a DNA repair enzyme; the **ERCC3 gene,** located on chromosome 2q21, which encodes for TFIIH basal transcription factor complex helicase; the **XPC gene,** located on chromosome 3p25, which encodes for a DNA repair enzyme; the **ERCC2 gene,** located on chromosome 19q13.2, which encodes for TFIIH basal transcription factor complex helicase; the **DDB2 gene,** located on chromosome 11p12, which encodes for DNA damage binding protein 2; the **ERCC4 gene,** located on chromosome 16p13.3, which encodes for a DNA repair enzyme; and the **ERCC5 gene,** located on chromosome 13q33, which encodes for a DNA repair enzyme. There is an XP variant gene **(XPV gene or hRAD30 gene),** which encodes for DNA polymerase eta, which is involved in error-free replication of DNA damaged by UV radiation.

B. **Ataxia-telangiectasia (AT)** is an autosomal recessive genetic disorder involving a gene locus on chromosome 11q22-q23 in which the affected individuals are hypersensitive to **ionizing radiation.** AT is characterized by: cerebellar ataxia with depletion of Purkinje cells; progressive nystagmus; slurred speech; oculocutaneous telangiectasia initially in the bulbar conjunctiva followed by ear, eyelid, cheeks, and neck; immunodeficiency; and death in the second decade of life. AT is caused by genetic defects in **DNA recombination repair enzymes.** The **ATM gene (AT Mutated)** is involved in the cause of AT. The ATM gene located on chromosome 11q22 encodes for a protein where one region resembles a **PI-3 kinase** (phosphatidylinositol-3 kinase) and another region resembles a **DNA repair enzyme/cell-cycle checkpoint protein.**

C. **Fanconi anemia** (FA; the most common form of congenital aplastic anemia) is an autosomal recessive genetic disorder involving gene loci on chromosomes 16q24, 9q22, and 3p26 in which affected individuals are hypersensitive to **DNA cross-linking agents.** FA is characterized by short stature, hypopigmented spots, café-au-lait spots, hypogonadism, microcephaly, hypoplastic or aplastic thumbs, renal malformations including unilateral aplasia or horseshoe kidney, acute leukemia, progressive aplastic anemia, head and neck tumors, and medulloblastoma. FA is caused by genetic defects in **DNA recombination repair enzymes** used to repair chromosome defects that occur during homologous recombination. There are 11 complementation groups in FA **(FA-A to FA-L).** To date, 8 of the genes have been cloned. The **FA-A gene** (involved in 65% of FA cases), located on chromosome 16q24, encodes for a protein that normalizes cell growth, corrects sensitivity to chromosomal breakage in the presence of mitomycin C, and generally promotes genomic stability. Several of the FA genes form a nuclear-protein complex that interacts with **BRCA1 and BRCA2** (breast cancer susceptibility genes 1 and 2) as the final common pathway. In this regard, BRCA2 has been found to be identical to FANC-D1.

D. Bloom syndrome (BS) is an autosomal recessive genetic disorder involving a gene locus on chromosome 15q26 in which affected individuals are hypersensitive to a **wide variety of DNA-damaging agents.** BS is characterized by long, narrow face, erythema with telangiectasias in butterfly distribution over the nose and cheeks, high-pitched voice, small stature, small mandible, immunodeficiency with decreased IgA, IgM, and IgG levels, predisposition to several types of cancers, and increased frequency in the Ashkenazi Jewish population. BS is caused by genetic defects in enzymes involved in DNA repair. The **BLM gene** is involved in the cause of BS. The BLM gene located on chromosome 15q26 encodes for a protein that has strong homology to the **RecQ helicases** (a subfamily of DExH box-containing DNA and RNA helicases).

E. Hereditary nonpolyposis colorectal cancer (HNPCC) is an autosomal dominant genetic disorder that accounts for 3–5% of all colorectal cancers. HNPCC is characterized by onset at a young age, high frequency of carcinomas proximal to the splenic flexure, multiple synchronous or metachronous colorectal cancers, and the presence of extracolonic cancers (e.g., endometrial and ovarian cancer; adenocarcinomas of the stomach, small intestine, and hepatobiliary tract). HNPCC is caused by genetic defects in **DNA mismatch repair enzymes,** which recognize single nucleotide mismatches or loops that occur in microsatellite repeat areas. The **MLH1, MSH2, MSH6, PMS1, and PMS2 gene**s are involved in the cause of HPNCC. These genes are the human homologues to the *Escherichia coli* **mutS** and **mutL** genes, which code for DNA mismatch repair enzymes.

Ⓥ Selected Photographs

A. Chromosome 4p deletion (Wolf-Hirschhorn syndrome)and chromosome 5p deletion (cri-du-chat syndrome) (Figure 22-1A and B)

B. Prader-Willi syndrome, Angelman syndrome, DiGeorge syndrome, Miller-Dieker syndrome (Figure 22-2 A–D)

C. Robertsonian t(13q14q), Robertsonian t(14q21q), acute promyelocytic leukemia t(15;17)(q21;q21), chronic myeloid leukemia t(9;22)(q34;q11) (Figure 22-3 A–D)

D. Fragile X syndrome, xeroderma pigmentosum, ataxia-telangiectasia, Fanconi anemia, Bloom syndrome (Figure 22-4A–E)

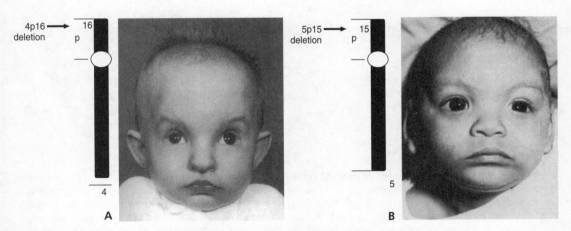

● **Figure 22.1 Deletion abnormalities. (A)** Chromosome 4p deletion (Wolf-Hirschhorn syndrome). The deletion at 4p16 is shown on chromosome 4. A photograph of a 5-year-old boy with Wolf-Hirschhorn syndrome showing a prominent forehead and broad nasal root ("Greek warrior helmet"), short philtrum, downturned mouth, and severe mental retardation (IQ of 20). **(B)** Chromosome 5p deletion (cri-du-chat or cat-cry syndrome). The deletion at 5p15 is shown on chromosome 5. A photograph of an infant with cri-du-chat showing round facies, microcephaly, and mental retardation.

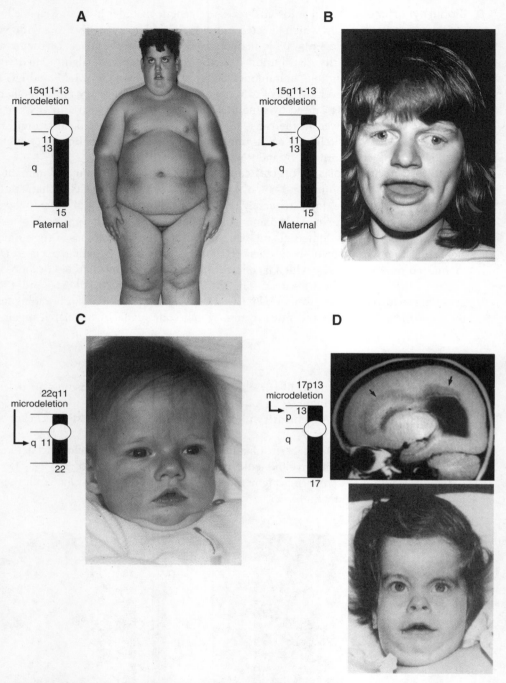

● Figure 22.2 Microdeletion abnormalities. (A) Prader-Willi syndrome. The microdeletion at 15q11-13 is shown on chromosome 15, inherited from the father (paternal). A photograph of a 10-year-old boy with Prader-Willi syndrome showing hypogonadism, hypotonia, obesity, short stature, and small hands and feet. **(B)** Angelman syndrome ("happy puppet" syndrome). The microdeletion at 15q11-13 is shown on chromosome 15, inherited from the mother (maternal). A photograph of a young woman with Angelman syndrome showing a happy disposition with inappropriate laughter and severe mental retardation (only 5- to 10-word vocabulary). **(C)** DiGeorge syndrome. The microdeletion at 22q11 is shown on chromosome 22. A photomicrograph of a lymph node from a patient with DiGeorge syndrome showing the absence of T lymphocytes within the inner cortex (IC; or paracortex; or thymic-dependent zone). The outer cortex (OC) shows abundant B lymphocytes within lymphatic follicles. **(D)** Miller-Dieker syndrome (agyria, lissencephaly). The microdeletion at 17p13.3 is shown on chromosome 17. MRI (top figure) shows a complete absence of gyri in the cerebral hemispheres. The lateral ventricles are indicated by the arrows. A photograph of a brain at autopsy from an infant with Miller-Dieker syndrome showing the complete absence of gyri.

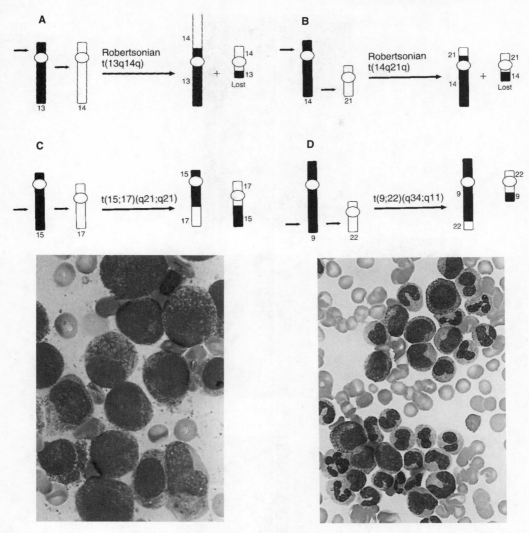

● **Figure 22.3 Translocation abnormalities. (A)** Robertsonian t(13q14q). **(B)** Robertsonian t(14q21q). **(C)** Acute promyelocytic leukemia t(15;17)(q21;q21). The translocation between chromosomes 15 and 17 is shown. A photomicrograph of acute promyelocytic leukemia showing abnormal promyelocytes with their characteristic pattern of heavy granulation and bundle of Auer rods. **(D)** Chronic myeloid leukemia t(9;22)(q34;q11). The translocation between chromosomes 9 and 22 is shown. A photomicrograph of chronic myeloid leukemia showing marker granulocytic hyperplasia with neutrophilic precursors at all stages of maturation. Erythroid (red blood cell) precursors are significantly decreased, with none shown in this field.

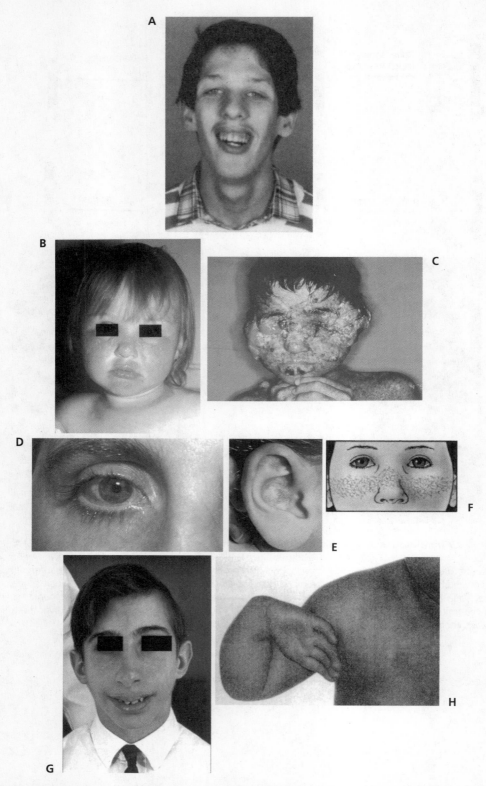

● **Figure 22.4 Fragile site and breakage abnormalities. (A)** Fragile-X syndrome. **(B,C)** Xeroderma pigmentosum. **(D–F)** Ataxia-telangiectasia. **(G)** Fanconi syndrome. **(H)** Bloom syndrome.

Chapter 23

Single-Gene Inherited Diseases

I. Autosomal Dominant Inheritance

A. Introduction. In autosomal dominant inheritance, the disease is observed **in both males and females with equal probability** who are *heterozygous for the mutant gene.* The characteristic pedigree is **vertical** in that the disease is passed from one generation to the next. An example of an autosomal dominant inherited disease is Huntington disease (HD).

B. Huntington disease (HD). HD involves a 26–100+ unstable repeat sequence of $(CAG)_n$ located in an exon (or coding) sequence of the HD gene on chromosome 4p16.3. HD is an autosomal dominant genetic disorder caused by the CAG repeat sequence on chromosome 4p16.3. The HD gene encodes for a protein called **huntingtin,** which is a cytoplasmic protein present in neurons within the striatum, cerebral cortex, and cerebellum, although its precise function is unknown. A primary manifestation is movement jerkiness most apparent at movement termination. HD is also characterized by: chorea (dance-like movements), memory deficits, affective disturbances, personality changes, diffuse and marked atrophy of the neostriatum due to cell death of cholinergic neurons and GABA-ergic neurons within the striatum (caudate nucleus and putamen) and a relative increase in dopaminergic neuron activity, and neuronal intranuclear aggregates.

II. Autosomal Recessive Inheritance

A. Introduction. In autosomal recessive inheritance, the disease is observed **in both males and females with equal probability** who are *homozygous for the mutant gene.* The characteristic pedigree is **horizontal,** in that affected individuals tend to be limited to a single sibship and the disease is not found in multiple generations. An example of an autosomal recessive inherited disease is cystic fibrosis (CF). Other autosomal recessive inherited disorders are listed in Table 23-1.

B. Cystic fibrosis (CF). CF is characterized by the **production of abnormally thick mucus** by epithelial cells lining the respiratory and gastrointestinal tracts. This results clinically in **obstruction of pulmonary airways** and **recurrent respiratory bacterial infections.** CF is caused by an **autosomal recessive** mutation such that an individual must receive two defective copies of the CF gene (one from each parent) to have the disease. The CF gene is located on the **long arm (q arm) of chromosome 7 (7q)** between bands q21 and q31. The CF gene encodes for a protein called **CFTR** (**c**ystic **f**ibrosis **tr**ansporter), which functions as a **Cl^- ion channel.** A mutation in the CF gene destroys the Cl^- transport function of CFTR. In North America, 70% of cystic fibrosis cases are due to a **three-base deletion** that codes for the amino acid **phenylalanine at position 508,** such that phenylalanine is missing from CFTR.

X-Linked Dominant Inheritance

A. Introduction. In X-linked dominant inheritance, the disease is observed **in both males and females (with no male-to-male transmission).** All daughters of an affected man will be affected because all receive the X chromosome bearing the mutant gene from their father. All sons of an affected man will be normal because they receive only the Y chromosome from the father. An example of an X-linked dominant inherited disease is hypophosphatemic rickets. Other X-linked dominant inherited disorders are listed in Table 23-1.

B. Hypophosphatemic rickets (HR). HR is a vitamin D–resistant rickets characterized by low blood PO_4^{2-} levels, high urinary PO_4^{2-} levels, short stature, and bony deformities.

 X-Linked Recessive Inheritance

A. Introduction. In X-linked recessive inheritance, the disease is *usually* observed **only in the males (with no male-to-male transmission),** since males have only one X chromosome; that is, males are **hemizygous** for X-linked genes (i.e., there is no backup copy of the gene). In X-linked recessive inheritance, heterozygous females are clinically normal but may be detected by subtle clinical features (like intermediate enzyme levels, etc.). Can the disease ever be observed in females? The answer is yes according the following mechanism: In females, one of the two X chromosomes is inactivated during the **late blastocyst stage** to form a **Barr body** in a process called **dosage compensation (or lyonization).** The choice of whether the maternally derived or paternally derived X chromosome gets inactivated is a **random** and **permanent event.** The mechanism of dosage compensation involves **methylation of cytosine nucleotides.** If the X chromosome with the normal gene is inactivated, the female has one X chromosome with the abnormal gene and will therefore be affected by the disease. An example of X-linked recessive inherited disease is Duchenne muscular dystrophy (DMD). Other X-linked recessive inherited disorders are listed in Table 23-1.

B. Duchenne muscular dystrophy (DMD). DMD is characterized by **progressive muscle weakness and wasting.** This results clinically in **premature death due to cardiac or respiratory failure** in the late teens to twenties. DMD is caused by an **X-linked recessive** mutation such that the male need receive only one defective copy of the DMD gene (from the mother) to have the disease. The DMD gene is located on the **short arm (p arm) of chromosome X in band 21 (Xp21).** The DMD gene encodes for a protein called **dystrophin,** which anchors the cytoskeleton (actin) of skeletal muscle cells to the extracellular matrix via a transmembrane protein (**α-dystrophin and β-dystrophin**), thereby stabilizing the cell membrane. A mutation of the DMD gene destroys the ability of dystrophin to anchor actin to the extracellular matrix.

Mitochondrial Inheritance

A. Introduction. In mitochondrial inheritance, the disease is observed in **both males and females who have an affected mother** (not father). Diseases that have mitochondrial inheritance are caused by mutations in the mitochondrial DNA (mtDNA). They are inherited entirely through **maternal transmission** because sperm mitochondria do not pass into the ovum at fertilization. Because mtDNA replicates autonomously from nuclear DNA and mitochondria segregate in daughter cells independently of nuclear chromosomes, the proportion of mitochondria carrying an mtDNA mutation can differ among somatic cells. This heterogeneity is termed **heteroplasmy** and plays a role in the variable phenotype of mitochondrial disease. An example of a mitochondrial inherited disease is Leber hereditary optic neuropathy (LHON). Other mitochondrial inherited disorders are listed in Table 23-1.

TABLE 23-1

A PARTIAL LIST OF INHERITED DISEASES BY TYPE

Autosomal Dominant	Autosomal Recessive	X-linked	Mitochondrial	Multifactorial
Achondroplasia	α_1-Antitrypsin deficiency	**Recessive**	Cardiac rhythm disturbances?	Cancer
Acrocephalosyndactyly	Adrenogenital syndromes	Duchenne muscular	Cardiomyopathies?	Cleft lip
Adult polycystic kidney	Albinism	dystrophy	Infantile bilateral striated	Cleft palate
disease	Alpha thalassemia	Ectodermal dysplasia	necrosis	Clubfoot
Alport syndrome	Alkaptonuria	Ehlers-Danlos (type IX)	Kearns-Sayre syndrome	Congenital heart defects
Apert syndrome	Argininosuccinic aciduria	Fabry disease	Leber hereditary optic	Coronary artery disease
Bor syndrome	Ataxia telangiectasia	Fragile X syndrome	neuropathy	Epilepsy
Brachydactyly	Beta thalassemia	G6PD deficiency		Hemochromatosis
Charcot-Marie-Tooth	Bloom syndrome	Hemophilia A and B		Hirschsprung disease
disease	Branched-chain ketonuria	Hunter syndrome		Hyperlipoproteinemia (types
Cleidocranial dysplasia	Childhood polycystic kidney	Ichthyosis		I, IIb, III, IV, V)
Crouzon craniofacial	disease	Kennedy syndrome		Hypertension
dysplasia	Cystic fibrosis	Kinky hair syndrome		Legg-Calvé-Perthes disease
Craniostenosis	Cystinuria	Lesch-Nyhan syndrome		Pyloric stenosis
Diabetes associated with	Dwarfism	Testicular feminization		Rheumatic fever
defects in genes for	Ehlers-Danlos syndrome	Wiskott-Aldrich syndrome		Type 1 diabetes (associated
glucokinase, HNF-1α,	(type VI)	**Dominant**		with islet cell antibodies)
and HNF-4α	Erythropoietic porphyria	Goltz syndrome		Type 2 diabetes (associated
Ehlers-Danlos syndrome	Fanconi anemia	Hypophosphatemic rickets		with insulin resistance
(type IV)	Friedreich ataxia	Incontinentia pigmenti		and obesity)
Epidermolysis bullosa	Fructosuria	Orofaciodigital syndrome		
simplex	Galactosemia			
Familial adenomatous	Glycogen storage disease			
polyposis	Von Gierke (type Ia)			
Familial	Pompe (type II)			
hypercholesterolemia	Cori (type IIIa)			
(type IIa)	Andersen (type IV)			
Goldenhar syndrome	McArdle (type V)			
Heart-hand syndrome	Hers (type VI)			
Hereditary nonpolyposis	Tarui (type VIII)			
colorectal cancer	Hemoglobin C disease			
(HNPCC)	Hepatolenticular			
Hereditary spherocytosis	degeneration			

Continued

TABLE 23-1

A PARTIAL LIST OF INHERITED DISEASES BY TYPE (CONTINUED)

Autosomal Dominant	Autosomal Recessive	X-linked	Mitochondrial	Multifactorial
Huntington disease	Histidinemia			
Marfan syndrome	Homocystinuria			
Monilethrix	Hypophosphatasia			
Myotonic dystrophy 1 and 2	Hypothyroidism			
Neurofibromatosis	Junctional epidermolysis bullosa			
Noonan syndrome	Juvenile myoclonic epilepsy			
Osteogenesis imperfecta (types I and IV)	Lawrence-Moon syndrome			
Pfeiffer syndrome	Lysosomal storage diseases			
Piebaldism	Tay Sachs			
Retinoblastoma	Gaucher			
Spinocerebellar ataxia 1, 2, 3, 6, 7, 8, 11, 17	Niemann-Pick			
Treacher Collins syndrome	Krabbe			
Uncombable hair syndrome	Sandhoff			
Von Willebrand disease	Schindler			
Waardenburg syndrome	GM_1 gangliosidosis			
Williams-Beuren syndrome	Metachromatic leukodystrophy			
	Mucopolysaccharidoses			
	Hurler			
	Sanfilippo A–D			
	Morquio A and B			
	Maroteaux-Lamy			
	Sly			
	Osteogenesis imperfecta (types II and III)			
	Oculocutaneous albinism (types I and II)			
	Peroxisomal disorders			
	Phenylketonuria			
	Premature senility			
	Pyruvate kinase deficiency			
	Retinitis pigmentosa			
	Sickle cell anemia			
	Trichothiodystrophy			
	Tyrosinemia			
	Xeroderma pigmentosum			

B. **Leber hereditary optic neuropathy (LHON).** LHON is characterized by **progressive optic nerve degeneration.** This results clinically in **blindness.** LHON is due to mutations in **mitochondrial DNA (mtDNA)** such that the inheritance is entirely by **maternal transmission,** since mtDNA is inherited only from the mother (because sperm mitochondria do *not* pass into the ovum at fertilization). Some 50% of all cases of LHON involve the **ND4 gene,** located on mtDNA when a missense mutation changes an **arginine to histidine.** The ND4 gene encodes for a protein called **subunit 4 of the NADH dehydrogenase complex,** which functions in the **electron transport chain** and the **production of ATP.** A mutation of the ND4 gene decreases the production of ATP, such that the demands of a very active neuronal metabolism cannot be met.

VI ## The Family Pedigree in Various Inherited Diseases (**Figure 23-1**). A family pedigree is a graphic method of charting the family history using various symbols.

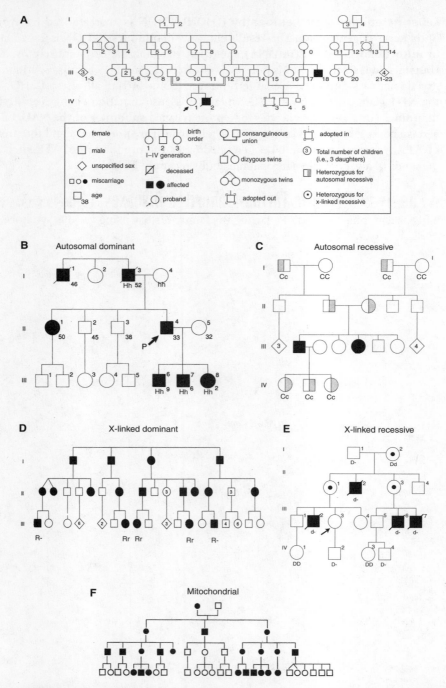

● **Figure 23.1 (A) A prototype family pedigree and explanation of the various symbols. (B) Pedigree of autoso-mal dominant inheritance.** The disease is observed in both males and females who are *heterozygous for the mutant gene* with equal probability. The characteristic pedigree is vertical in that the disease is passed from one generation to the next. **(C) Pedigree of autosomal recessive inheritance.** The disease is observed in both males and females who are *homozygous for the mutant gene* with equal probability. The characteristic pedigree is horizontal in that affected individuals tend to be limited to a single sibship and the disease is not found in multiple generations. **(D) Pedigree of X-linked domi-nant inheritance.** The disease is observed in both males and females (with no male-to-male transmission). All daughters of an affected man will be affected because all receive the X chromosome bearing the mutant gene from their father. All sons of an affected man will be normal because they receive only the Y chromosome from the father. **(E) Pedigree of X-linked recessive inheritance.** The disease is *usually* observed only in the males (with no male-to-male transmission). **(F) Pedigree of mitochondrial inheritance.** The disease is observed in both males and females who have an affected mother. Note that affected sons and daughters are siblings of an affected mother, and affected fathers do not produce affected siblings.

Chapter 24

Multifactorial Inherited Diseases

I Introduction. Multifactorial inheritance involves many genes that have a small, equal, and additive effect **(genetic component)**; it also involves an **environmental component.** Both components contribute to a person's inheritance of the liability to develop a certain disease. If one considers only the genetic component of a multifactorial disease, the term **polygenic** is used. An example of a multifactorial disease is type 1 diabetes. Other multifactorial inherited disorders are listed in Table 23-1.

II Type 1 Diabetes. The characteristic dysfunction is a **destruction of pancreatic beta cells,** which produce insulin. This results clinically in hyperglycemia, ketoacidosis, and exogenous insulin dependence. Long-term clinical effects include neuropathy, retinopathy leading to blindness, and nephropathy leading to kidney failure. Type 1 diabetes demonstrates an association with the highly polymorphic **HLA (human leukocyte antigen) class II genes,** which play a role in immune responsiveness. The specific loci involved in type 1 diabetes are called **HLA-DR3** and **HLA-DR4 loci.** These loci are located on the **short arm (p arm) of chromosome 6 (p6).** HLA-DR3 and HLA-DR4 loci code for **cell-surface glycoproteins,** which are structurally similar to immunoglobulin proteins and are expressed mainly by B lymphocytes and macrophages. It is *hypothesized* that alleles closely linked to HLA-DR3 and HLA-DR4 loci somehow alter the immune response such that the individual has an immune response to an environmental antigen (e.g., a virus). The immune response "spills over" and leads to the destruction of pancreatic beta cells. Markers for immune destruction of pancreatic beta cells include **autoantibodies to glutamic acid decarboxylase (GAD_{65}), insulin,** and **tyrosine phosphatases IA-2 and IA-2β.** At present, it is not known whether the autoantibodies play a causative role in the destruction of the pancreatic beta cell or whether the autoantibodies form secondarily, after the pancreatic beta cells have been destroyed.

Chapter 25

Teratology

I Introduction. A teratogen is any infectious agent, drug, chemical, or irradiation that alters fetal morphology or fetal function if the fetus is exposed during a critical stage of development.

A. The **resistant period (week 1 of development)** is the time when the conceptus demonstrates the "all-or-none" phenomenon (i.e., the conceptus will either die as a result of the teratogen or survive unaffected).

B. The **maximum susceptibility period (weeks 3–8; embryonic period)** is the time when the embryo is most susceptible to teratogens, since all organ morphogenesis occurs at this time.

C. The **lowered susceptibility period (weeks 9–38; fetal period)** is the time when the fetus has a lowered susceptibility to teratogens, since all organ systems have already formed; exposure to a teratogen generally results in the *functional* derangement of an organ system.

II Infectious Agents may be viral or nonviral. However, bacteria appear to be nonteratogenic.

A. **Viral infections** may reach the fetus via the amniotic fluid following vaginal infection, transplacentally via the bloodstream after maternal viremia, or by direct contact during passage through an infected birth canal.

1. **Rubella virus (German measles, a member of TORCH)** belongs to the **Togaviridae** family, whose members are **enveloped, icosahedral, positive single-stranded RNA viruses.** The rubella virus is transmitted to the fetus **transplacentally.** The risk of fetal rubella infection is greatest during the **first month of pregnancy** and apparently declines thereafter. Fetal rubella infection results in the classic triad of **cardiac defects** (e.g., patent ductus arteriosus, pulmonary artery stenosis, atrioventricular (AV) septal defects), **cataracts,** and **low birth weight.** With the pandemic of rubella in 1964, the complexity of this syndrome became apparent and the term **"expanded rubella syndrome"** became standard. The clinical manifestations include intrauterine growth retardation (the most common manifestation), hepatosplenomegaly, generalized adenopathy, hemolytic anemia, hepatitis, jaundice, meningoencephalitis, eye involvement (e.g., cataracts, glaucoma, retinopathy), bluish-purple lesions on a yellow, jaundiced skin ("blueberry muffin" spots), osteitis (celery-stalk appearance of long bones), and sensorineural deafness. Exposure of a pregnant woman requires immediate assessment of her immune status. If the exposed woman is known to be immune (i.e., antibodies present), she can be assured of no risk. Postexposure prophylaxis of pregnant women with immune globulin (IG) is not recommended and should be considered only if abortion is not an option. Control measures for rubella prevention should be placed on immunization of children.

2. **Cytomegalovirus (CMV, a member of TORCH)** belongs to the **Herpesvirus** family, comprising **large, enveloped, icosahedral, double-stranded DNA viruses.** CMV is a ubiquitous virus and the **most common fetal infection.** CMV is transmitted to the fetus **transplacentally,** with more severe malformations when infection occurs during the first half of pregnancy. CMV is also transmitted to perinates **during passage through the birth canal or in breast milk,** but it causes no apparent disease. Both primary and recurrent infections of the mother can result in the transmission of CMV to the fetus. In mothers with recurrent infection, the presence of CMV antibodies does not prevent CMV transmission to the fetus but does protect the fetus from major fetal malformations. Consequently, the risk of major fetal malformations is much higher in infants of mothers who had a primary CMV infection during pregnancy compared with those who have had recurrent infections. The most common manifestation of CMV fetal infection is **sensorineural deafness. Cytomegalic inclusion disease** (characterized by multiorgan involvement) is the most serious but least common manifestation of CMV infection and results in: intrauterine growth retardation, microcephaly, chorioretinitis, hepatosplenomegaly, osteitis (celery-stalk appearance of long bones), discrete cerebral calcifications, mental retardation, heart block, and bluish-purple lesions on a yellow, jaundiced skin ("blueberry muffin" spots). **Ganciclovir** treatment of the neonate is being evaluated for symptomatic congenital CMV infection.

3. **Herpes simplex virus (HSV-1 and HSV-2, members of TORCH)** belongs to the **Herpesvirus** family, comprising **large, enveloped, icosahedral, double-stranded DNA viruses.** Most neonatal infections are caused by HSV-2 (75% of the cases). HSV-2 is transmitted to the fetus **transplacentally** only occasionally (5% of the cases). HSV-2 is most commonly transmitted to the fetus by **direct contact during passage through an infected birth canal** (intrapartum; 85% of cases). The risk of neonatal infection is higher with primary maternal HSV infection (30%–50%) than with recurrent maternal HSV infection (3%) because the infant is exposed to large amounts of virus in the absence of neutralizing antibodies. **At 10–11 days of age,** some intrapartum HSV-infected infants present with the disease localized to the **skin** (discrete vesicular lesion, large bullae, or denuded skin; hallmark signs), **eye** (keratoconjunctivitis, uveitis, chorioretinitis, cataracts, retinal dysplasia), or **mouth** (ulcerative lesions of the mouth, tongue, or palate). **At 15–17 days of age,** some intrapartum HSV-infected infants present with **CNS involvement** (with or without skin, eye, or mouth involvement) due to axonal retrograde transport of HSV to the brain. Clinical manifestations of CNS involvement include lethargy, bulging fontanelles, focal or generalized seizures, opisthotonos, decerebrate posturing, and coma. If the disease is untreated, there is a 40%–50% mortality rate and most survivors have neurologic sequelae. **At 9–11 days of age,** some intrapartum HSV-infected infants present with **disseminated disease.** Clinical manifestations of disseminated disease include CNS, liver, adrenal gland, pancreas, and kidney involvement due to hematogenous spread of HSV. If the disease is untreated, there is an 80% mortality rate and most survivors have neurologic sequelae. The only intervention shown to prevent neonatal HSV infection is delivery by cesarean section within 4–6 hours of rupture of the amnionic membranes. **Acyclovir suppressive therapy** has been used in women following a first episode of genital HSV infection during pregnancy to prevent a clinical HSV recurrence at delivery. The efficacy of acyclovir and valacyclovir treatment of the neonate is under study.

4. **Varicella zoster virus (VZV; varicella or chickenpox)** belongs to the **Herpesvirus** family, comprising **large, enveloped, icosahedral double-stranded DNA viruses.** VZV is the etiology of two clinical syndromes: a **primary infection** (varicella or chickenpox, which usually occurs in children) and a **secondary infection** (herpes zoster or shingles, which usually occurs in adults along a single sensory dermatome).

VZV is transmitted to the fetus **transplacentally** in 25% of the cases, but **fetal varicella syndrome** develops only when maternal VZV infection occurs in the first trimester. The clinical manifestations of fetal varicella syndrome include cicatricial (scarring) skin lesions in a dermatomal pattern, limb and digit hypoplasia, limb paresis/paralysis, hydrocephalus, microcephaly/mental retardation, seizures, chorioretinitis, and cataracts. Neonates whose mothers develop chickenpox 6–21 days before delivery do not show signs of severe chickenpox because maternal antibodies are produced and delivered to the fetus. Neonates whose mothers develop chickenpox fewer than 5 days before delivery or 2 days postpartum develop severe chickenpox, with increased mortality and morbidity (i.e., fever, skin lesions, hemorrhagic rash, respiratory distress, and pneumonia). **Acyclovir** treatment of the neonate is recommended. Varicella zoster immunoglobulin (VZIG) is recommended for neonates whose mothers develop chickenpox fewer than 5 days before delivery or 2 days postpartum. Administration of the live, attenuated VZV vaccine to susceptible women *before* pregnancy and to their susceptible household members (older than 1 year) is the most effective method of prevention.

5. **Human immunodeficiency virus (HIV)** belongs to the **Retroviridae** family (or **Lentivirinae** subfamily), comprising **diploid, enveloped, positive single-stranded RNA viruses.** HIV is believed by many investigators to be the major cause **acquired immunodeficiency syndrome (AIDS).** However, others believe that multiple blood transfusions (e.g., as in hemophiliacs), consumption of megadoses of antibiotics as prophylaxis against sexually transmitted diseases, and continuous use of drugs to heighten orgasm (e.g., amyl and butyl nitrite) destroy $CD4^+$ T cells and lead to AIDS. The placenta is a highly effective barrier to HIV infection of the fetus. However, HIV is transmitted to the fetus **through blood containing HIV or HIV-infected lymphoid cells** near the time of delivery or after 35 weeks of gestation. Increased exposure of the fetus or neonate to maternal HIV-infected blood increases the risk of HIV transmission. HIV infection does not appear to cause any congenital malformations but results in chronic, multisystemic infections. The clinical manifestations include **fungal infections** (e.g., candidal esophagitis, cryptococcal meningitis, histoplasmosis, coccidioidomycosis, *Pneumocystis carinii* pneumonia), **bacterial infections** (e.g., *Mycobacterium tuberculosis, Mycobacterium avium–intracellulare* complex, *Streptococcus pneumoniae*, and gastroenteritis caused by *Salmonella, Shigella*, and *Campylobacter*), **viral infections** (e.g., HSV1, HSV2, and CMV), and protozoan infections (e.g., *Cryptosporidium, Giardia, Toxoplasma*, and *Entamoeba*). All HIV-infected children below 1 year of age should receive a regimen of two nucleoside reverse transcriptase (RT) inhibitors (e.g., zidovudine, didanosine, lamivudine, stavudine) and a nonnucleoside RT inhibitor (e.g., nevirapine, efavirenz) or a protease inhibitor (e.g., ritonavir, nelfinavir). Prevention of perinatal HIV transmission is accomplished by zidovudine treatment to the pregnant mother during pregnancy and to the newborn for the first 6 weeks of life.

B. **Nonviral infections**

1. **Toxoplasma gondii (TG; a member of TORCH)** is a **protozoan parasite** whose life cycle is divided into a **sexual phase** that occurs only in cats **(the definitive host)** and an **asexual phase** that occurs in intermediate hosts. Generally speaking, mice that eat cat feces contaminate fields, thereby infecting cows, sheep, and pigs. TG is transmitted to humans primarily through ingestion of oocyst-containing water or food or consumption of cyst-containing raw or undercooked meat. In addition, inhalation or ingestion of oocysts from soil, dust, or a cat litter box may occur. TG is transmitted to the fetus **transplacentally** in 25%, 54%, and 65% of pregnant women with untreated primary toxoplasmosis during the first, second, and third trimesters, respectively. TG infection results in miscarriage, perinatal death, chorioretinitis, mi-

crocephaly, hydrocephalus, and encephalomyelitis with cerebral calcification. About 10% of congenitally infected infants who have severe TG die, while most surviving infants are left with major neurologic sequelae (e.g., mental retardation, seizures, spasticity, and visual deficits). Acutely infected women who elect to proceed with the pregnancy should be treated with **spiramycin** (a macrolide antibiotic). If prenatal diagnosis indicates that the fetus is infected, then **pyrimethamine** (a folic acid antagonist), **sulfadiazine** (a folic acid antagonist), and **leucovorin** (folinic acid) are added.

2. *Treponema pallidum* **(TP)** is the **spirochete** causing **syphilis** and is transmitted to the fetus **transplacentally** in 10%, 40%, 50%, and 50% of pregnant women with a late latent stage, early latent stage, primary stage, and secondary stage of syphilis, respectively. Infection acquired at birth through contact with a genital lesion in the birth canal may also occur but is rare. The most important determinant of risk to the fetus is the maternal stage of syphilis. TP infection results in miscarriage; perinatal death; hepatosplenomegaly; hepatitis; joint swelling; vesiculobullous blisters, whose fluid contains active spirochetes and is highly infective; nasal discharge with rhinitis; a maculopapular rash located on the extremities, which is initially oval and pink but then turns copper-brown and desquamates (palms and soles; eye findings include chorioretinitis, glaucoma, cataracts, and uveitis); anemia; jaundice; focal erosions of the proximal medial tibia (Wimberger sign); osteitis (celery-stalk appearance of long bones); sawtooth appearance of the metaphyses of long bones; abnormal teeth (Hutchinson teeth); acute syphilitic leptomeningitis, which may present as neck stiffness; and chronic meningovascular syphilis (cranial nerve palsy, hydrocephalus, cerebral infarction). **"Early congenital syphilis"** refers to those clinical manifestations that appear **within 2 years of age.** **"Late congenital syphilis"** refers to those clinical manifestations that appear **after 2 years of age.** Some infants may remain asymptomatic until 2–5 years of age. The clinical manifestations of late congenital syphilis result from the inflammation of scars caused by early congenital syphilis. Penicillin treatment given to the infected mother usually provides adequate therapy for the fetus. If not, the infant is treated with penicillin. All pregnant women should be tested for syphilis on their first antenatal visit. For high-risk women, additional tests at 28 weeks of gestation and at delivery should be performed.

III **TORCH Infections.** These infections are caused by *Toxoplasma* **(T)**, **rubella (R)**, **cytomegalovirus (C)**, **herpesvirus (H)**, and **other (O)** bacterial and viral infections, which are grouped together because they cause similar clinical and pathologic manifestations. See above discussion for specifics.

IV **Childhood Vaccinations.** A general practical guide to childhood vaccinations includes the following:

A. **MMR** vaccine given in two doses at 12–15 months and at 4–6 years protects against **m**easles, **m**umps, and **r**ubella.

B. **Polio vaccine** protects against polio given in four doses at 2 months, 4 months, 6–18 months, and 4–6 years.

C. **DTaP vaccine** protects against **d**iphtheria, **t**etanus, and **p**ertussis given in five doses at 2 months, 4 months, 6 months, 15–18 months, and 4–6 years. A tetanus booster is given at 11 years.

D. **Hib vaccine** protects against *Haemophilus influenzae type b* given in four doses at 2 months, 4 months, 6 months, and 12–15 months.

E. **HBV vaccine** protects against **h**epatitis **B** **v**irus given in four doses at birth, 1 month, 4 months, and 6–18 months.

F. **Varicella vaccine** protects against chicken pox given in one dose at 12–18 months.

G. **Pneumococcal vaccine (PCV7)** protects against pneumonia, blood infections, and meninigitis in four doses at 2 months, 4 months, 6 months, and 12–25 months.

Ⓥ Category X Drugs (Absolute Contraindication in Pregnancy)

A. **Thalidomide** is an **antinauseant** drug that was prescribed for pregnant women (no longer used) for "morning sickness." This drug can cause: limb reduction (e.g., meromelia, amelia), ear and nasal abnormalities, cardiac defects, lung defects, pyloric or duodenal stenosis, and gastrointestinal atresia.

B. **Aminopterin and methotrexate** are **folic acid antagonists** used in cancer chemotherapy. These drugs can cause: small stature, abnormal cranial ossification, ocular hypertelorism, low-set ears, cleft palate, and myelomeningocele.

C. **Busulfan (Myleran), chlorambucil (Leukeran), cyclophosphamide (Cytoxan)** are **alkylating agents** used in cancer chemotherapy. These drugs can cause: cleft palate, eye defects, hydronephrosis, renal agenesis, absence of toes, and growth retardation.

D. **Phenytoin (Dilantin)** is an **antiepileptic** drug. In 30% of cases, this drug causes: **fetal hydantoin syndrome,** which results in growth retardation, mental retardation, microcephaly, craniofacial defects, and nail and digit hypoplasia. In the majority of cases, this drug causes cleft lip, cleft palate, and congenital heart defects.

E. **Triazolam (Halcion) and estazolam (ProSom)** are **hypnotic** drugs. These drugs can cause cleft lip and cleft palate, especially if used in the first trimester of pregnancy.

F. **Warfarin (Coumadin)** is an **anticoagulant** drug that acts by inhibiting vitamin K–dependent coagulation factors. This drug can cause stippled epiphyses, mental retardation, microcephaly, seizures, fetal hemorrhage, and optic atrophy in the fetus. Note the mnemonic *war*farin serves as a reminder of WAR in the fetus.

G. **Isotretinoin (Accutane)** is a **retinoic acid derivative** used in the treatment of **severe acne.** This drug can cause CNS abnormalities, external ear abnormalities, eye abnormalities, facial dysmorphia, and cleft palate (i.e., **vitamin A embryopathy**).

H. **Clomiphene (Clomid)** is a nonsteroidal **ovulatory stimulant** used in women with ovulatory dysfunction. Although no causative evidence of a deleterious effect of clomiphene on the human fetus has been established, there have been reports of birth anomalies.

I. **Diethylstilbestrol** is a **synthetic estrogen** that was used in the past to prevent spontaneous abortion in women. This drug can cause cervical hood, T-shaped uterus, hypoplastic uterus, ovulatory disorders, infertility, premature labor, and cervical incompetence in women who were exposed to DES in utero. These women are also subject to an increased risk of adenocarcinoma of the vagina later in life.

J. **Ethisterone, norethisterone, and megestrol (Megace)** are synthetic **progesterone derivatives.** These drugs can cause masculinization of genitalia in female embryos, hypospadias in males, and cardiovascular anomalies.

K. **Ovcon, Levlen, and Norinyl** are **oral contraceptives** that contain a combination of estrogen (e.g., ethinyl estradiol or mestranol) and progesterone (e.g., norethindrone or levonorgestrel) derivatives. These drugs can cause an increase of fetal abnormalities, particularly the **VACTERL syndrome,** consisting of **v**ertebral, **a**nal, **c**ardiac, **t**racheoe**s**ophageal, **r**enal, and **l**imb malformations.

L. **Nicotine** is a **poisonous, addictive alkaloid** delivered to the fetus through **cigarette smoking** by pregnant women (cigarette smoke also contains **hydrogen cyanide** and **carbon monoxide**). This drug can cause intrauterine growth retardation, premature delivery, low birth weight, and fetal hypoxia due to reduced uterine blood flow and diminished capacity of the blood to transport oxygen to fetal tissue.

M. **Alcohol** is an **organic compound** delivered to the fetus through **recreational or addictive (i.e., alcoholism) drinking** by pregnant women. This drug can cause **fetal alcohol syndrome,** which results in mental retardation, microcephaly, holoprosencephaly, limb deformities, craniofacial abnormalities (i.e., hypertelorism, long philtrum, and short palpebral fissures), and cardiovascular defects (i.e., ventricular septal defects). Fetal alcohol syndrome is the leading cause of mental retardation.

VI # Category D Drugs (Definite Evidence of Risk to Fetus)

A. **Tetracycline (Achromycin) and doxycycline (Vibramycin)** are **antibiotics** in the tetracycline family. These drugs can cause permanently stained teeth and hypoplasia of enamel.

B. **Streptomycin, amikacin, and tobramycin (Nebcin)** are **antibiotics** in the aminoglycoside family. These drugs can cause **CN VIII toxicity,** with permanent bilateral deafness and loss of vestibular function.

C. **Phenobarbital (Donnatal) and pentobarbital (Nembutal)** are **barbiturates** used as **sedatives.** Studies have suggested a higher incidence of fetal abnormalities with maternal barbiturate use.

D. **Valproic acid (Depakene)** is an **antiepileptic** drug. It can cause neural tube defects, cleft lip, and renal defects.

E. **Diazepam (Valium), chlordiazepoxide (Librium), alprazolam (Xanax), and lorazepam (Ativan)** are **anticonvulsant** and **antianxiety** drugs. These drugs can cause cleft lip and cleft palate, especially if used in the first trimester of pregnancy.

F. **Lithium** is used in the treatment of **manic-depressive disorder.** This drug can cause fetal cardiac defects (i.e., Ebstein anomaly and malformations of the great vessels).

G. **Chlorothiazide (Diuril)** is a **diuretic** and **antihypertensive** drug. This drug can cause fetal jaundice and thrombocytopenia.

VII # Chemical Agents

A. **Organic mercury.** Consumption of organic mercury during pregnancy results in fetal neurologic damage, including seizures, psychomotor retardation, cerebral palsy, blindness, and deafness.

B. **Lead.** Consumption of lead during pregnancy results in abortion due to embryotoxicity, growth retardation, increased perinatal mortality, and developmental delay.

C. **Polychlorinated biphenyls (PCBs).** Consumption of PCBs during pregnancy results in intrauterine growth retardation, dark-brown skin pigmentation, exophthalmos, gingival hyperplasia, skull calcification, mental retardation, and neurobehavioral abnormalities.

D. **Bisphenol A** is a common ingredient in plastics used to make reusable water bottles and in resins used to line food cans and dental sealants. Bisphenol A has been associated with higher rates of breast cancer in animal studies.

E. **Phthalates** are a common ingredient in vinyl flooring, detergents, automotive plastics, soap, shampoo, deodorants, hair sprays, blood storage bags, and intravenous medical tubing. High phthalate levels in pregnant women have been associated with testicular changes in their infant sons, leading to lower concentrations of male hormones and incomplete testicular descent. Phthalates have antiandrogenic activity.

F. **Perfluorooctanoic acid (PFOA)** is a common ingredient of stain-, grease-, and water-resistant plastics like Teflon and Gore-Tex. PFOA is a likely carcinogen associated with liver, breast, pancreatic, and testicular cancers.

G. **Methoxychlor (an insecticide) and vinclozolin (a fungicide)** are considered "endocrine disruptors." Recent studies have shown that the exposure of pregnant mice to either of these chemicals affected not just the male offspring exposed in utero but all males for the four subsequent generations.

H. Potassium iodide (PI). PI is found in over-the-counter cough medicines and radiograph cocktails for organ visualization. PI is involved in: thyroid enlargement (goiter) and mental retardation (cretinism).

VIII Recreational Drugs

A. **Lysergic acid diethylamide (LSD)** has not been shown to be teratogenic.
B. **Marijuana** has not been shown to be teratogenic.
C. **Caffeine** has not been shown to be teratogenic.
D. **Cocaine** results in an increased risk of various congenital abnormalities, stillbirth, low birth weight, and placental abruption.
E. **Heroin** has not been shown to be teratogenic. It is the drugs that are often taken *with* heroin that produce congenital anomalies. The principal adverse effect is **severe neonatal withdrawal,** causing death in 3–5% of neonates. **Methadone** (used to replace heroin) is not teratogenic but is also associated with severe neonatal withdrawal.

IX Ionizing Radiation

A. Exposure to **acute high doses (over 250 rads)** of ionizing radiation results in microcephaly, mental retardation, growth retardation, and leukemia. After exposure to **greater than 25 rads,** classic fetal defects will be observed, so that termination of pregnancy should be offered as an option. Much information concerning acute high-dose radiation exposure has come from studies of the atomic explosions over Hiroshima and Nagasaki.
B. **Diagnostic radiation.** Even if several radiographic studies are performed, the dose rarely adds up to exposure significant enough to produce fetal defects. **Radioactive iodine cocktails** for organ visualization should be avoided after week 10 of gestation, since fetal thyroid development can be impaired.

X Selected Photographs

A. **TORCH** (Figure 25-1)
B. **Neonatal syphilis** (Figure 25-2)

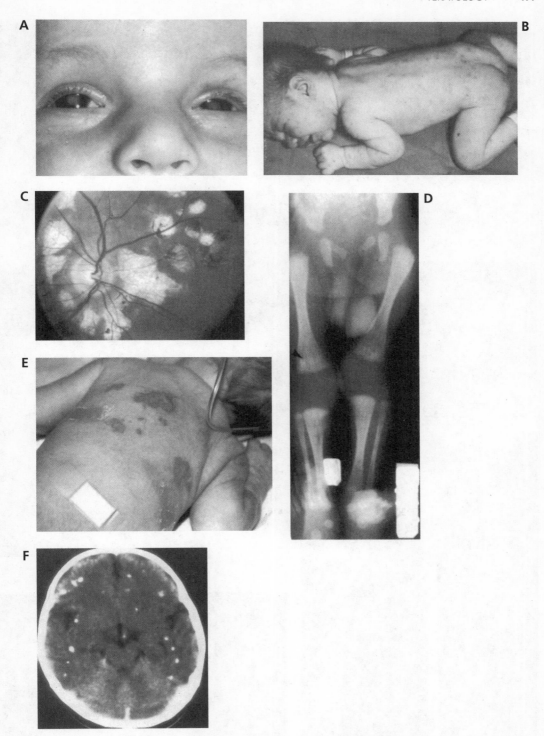

● **Figure 25.1 TORCH infections. (A)** Cataracts seen with congenital rubella and herpes simplex virus infections. **(B)** "Blueberry muffin" spots seen with congenital rubella and cytomegalovirus infections due to extramedullary hematopoiesis. **(C)** Patchy, yellow-white lesions of chorioretinitis seen with congenital cytomegalovirus, herpes simplex virus, and *Toxoplasma gondii* infections. **(D)** Celery-stalk appearance of the femur (arrowhead) and tibia seen with congenital rubella, cytomegalovirus, and syphilis infections. The alternating bands of longitudinal translucency and density indicate a disturbance in normal bone metabolism. **(E)** Cutaneous vesicular lesions surrounded by an erythematous border on the back and right arm seen with congenital herpes simplex virus infection. **(F)** Diffuse cerebral calcifications seen with congenital cytomegalovirus and *Toxoplasma gondii* infections.

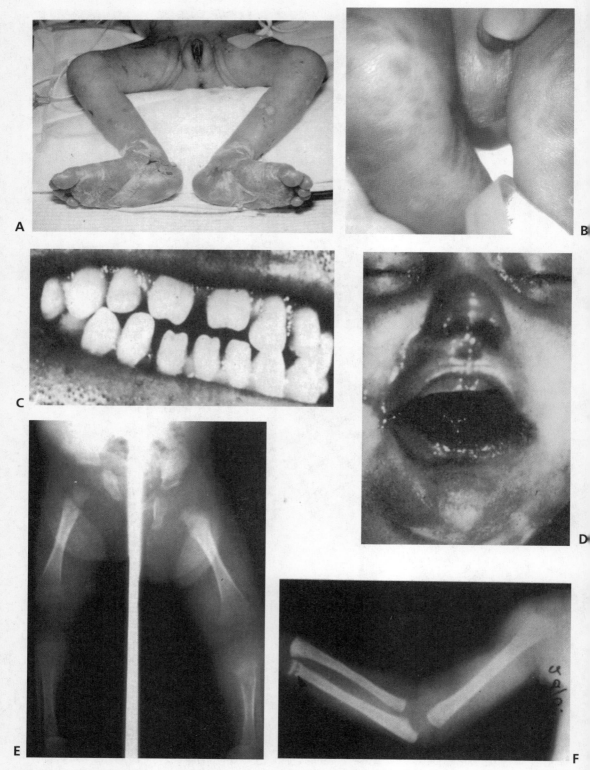

● **Figure 25.2 Congenital syphilis. (A)** Vesiculobullous blisters on the legs and feet (arrows) along with marked skin peeling. **(B)** A copper-brown rash on the extremities. **(C)** Hutchinson teeth, which are small, widely spaced, and have notched upper central incisors. **(D)** Nasal discharge with rhinitis. **(E)** The Wimberger sign shows focal erosions of the proximal medial tibia. **(F)** Sawtooth appearance of the distal radius. The radiolucent area represents syphilitic granulation tissue.

Credits

Figure 1-1: Adapted from Dudek RW, Fix JD. Board Review Series: Embryology. 2nd Ed. Philadelphia: Lippincott Williams & Wilkins, 1998:4.

Figure 1-2: From Dudek RW. High-Yield Histology. 2nd Ed. Philadelphia: Lippincott Williams & Wilkins, 2000:170.

Figure 3-2: From Sternberg SS. Diagnostic Surgical Pathology, vol 2, 3rd Ed. Philadelphia: Lippincott Williams & Wilkins, 1999.

Figure 4-2: From Dudek RW, Fix JD. Board Review Series: Embryology. 3rd Ed. Philadelphia: Lippincott Williams & Wilkins, 2005:27.

Figure 4-4: A,B. From Sadler TW. Langman's Medical Embryology. 7th Ed. Philadelphia: Lippincott Williams & Wilkins, 1995:62. **A.** Courtesy of Dr. Don Nakayama, Department of Surgery, University of North Carolina.

Figure 5-2: From Dudek RW, Fix JD. Board Review Series: Embryology. 3rd Ed. Philadelphia: Lippincott Williams & Wilkins, 2005:26.

Figure 5-3: From Dudek RW, Fix JD. Board Review Series: Embryology. 3rd Ed. Philadelphia: Lippincott Williams & Wilkins, 2005:54.

Figure 6-2: From Dudek RW, Fix JD. Board Review Series: Embryology. 3rd Ed. Philadelphia: Lippincott Williams & Wilkins, 2005:34.

Figure 6-3: From Dudek RW, Fix JD. Board Review Series: Embryology. 3rd Ed. Philadelphia: Lippincott Williams & Wilkins, 2005:36. **Radiograph in B.** From McMillan JA, DeAngelis CD, Feigin RD, et al., eds. Oski's Pediatrics. 3rd Ed. Philadelphia: Lippincott Williams & Wilkins, 1999:1349.

Figure 6-4: From Dudek RW, Fix JD. Board Review Series: Embryology. 3rd Ed. Philadelphia: Lippincott Williams & Wilkins, 2005:37. **Radiographs in B.** From Kirks DR, Griscom NT. Practical Pediatric Imaging. 3rd Ed. Philadelphia: Lippincott Williams & Wilkins, 1997:555.

Figure 6-5: From Dudek RW, Fix JD. Board Review Series: Embryology. 3rd Ed. Philadelphia: Lippincott Williams & Wilkins, 2005:38. **Radiographs in B.** From Kirks DR, Griscom NT. Practical Pediatric Imaging. 3rd Ed. Philadelphia: Lippincott Williams & Wilkins, 1997:519. **Ventriculograph in B.** From McMillan JA, DeAngelis CD, Feigin RD, et al., eds. Oski's Pediatrics. 3rd Ed. Philadelphia: Lippincott Williams & Wilkins, 1999:1356.

Figure 7-2: A,C,D. From Fenoglio-Preiser CM, Davis M, eds. Gastrointestinal Pathology: An Atlas and Text. 2nd Ed. Philadelphia: Lippincott Williams & Wilkins, 1998. **B.** From Fenoglio-Preiser CM, Davis M, eds. Gastrointestinal Pathology: An Atlas and Text. 2nd Ed. Philadelphia: Lippincott Williams & Wilkins, 1998. Courtesy of Dr. Cooley Butler, Scripps Memorial Hospital, La Jolla, CA. **E,F.** From Yamada T, Alpers DH, Laine L, et al., eds. Textbook of Gastroenterology, vol 1, 3rd Ed. Philadelphia: Lippincott Williams & Wilkins, 1999:1189.

Figure 7-3: A. From Johnson KE. NMS Human Developmental Anatomy. Baltimore: Williams & Wilkins, 1988:211. **B.** Fenoglio-Preiser CM, Noffsinger AE, Stemmermann GN, et al., eds. Gastrointestinal Pathology: An Atlas and Text. 2nd Ed. Philadelphia: Lippincott Williams & Wilkins, 1998:155. Courtesy of Dr. K. Bove, Children's Hospital Medical Center, Cincinnati, OH. **C.** From Yamada T, Alpers DH, Laine L, et al., eds. Textbook of Gastroenterology, vol 1, 3rd Ed. Philadelphia: Lippincott Williams & Wilkins, 1999:1337.

Figure 7-4: A. From Johnson KE. NMS Human Developmental Anatomy. Baltimore: Williams & Wilkins, 1988:215. **B.** From Yamada T, Alpers DH, Laine L, et al., eds. Textbook of Gastroenterology, vol 1, 3rd Ed. Philadelphia: Lippincott Williams & Wilkins, 1999:2250.

Figure 7-5: A. From Johnson KE. NMS Human Developmental Anatomy. Baltimore: Williams & Wilkins, 1989:215. **A(1).** From Henrikson RC, Kaye G, Mazurkiewicz J. NMS Histology. Baltimore: Williams & Wilkins, 1997:368. **B–D.** Modified from Cubilla AL, Fitzgerald PJ. Tumors of the exocrine pancreas. In: Hartmann WH, Sobin LH, eds. Atlas of Tumor Pathology. 2nd series, fascicle 19. Washington, DC: Armed Forces Institute of Pathology, 1984. **E.** From Yamada T, Alpers DH, Laine L, et al., eds. Textbook of Gastroenterology, vol 2, 3rd Ed. Philadelpha: Lippincott Williams & Wilkins, 1999:2118. Courtesy of Dr. Peter B. Cotton, Durham, NC. **F.** From Yamada T, Alpers DH, Laine L, eds. Atlas of Gastroenterology. 2nd Ed. Baltimore: Williams & Wilkins, 1995:458. Courtesy of Dr. J. Rode. **G.** From Misiewicz JJ, Bartram CI, Cotton PB, et al. Atlas of Clinical Gastroenterology. London: Gower Medical Publishing, 1987.

Figure 7-6: A. From Johnson KE. NMS Human Developmental Anatomy. Baltimore: Williams & Wilkins, 1988:218. **B,C.** From Sadler TW. Langman's Medical Embryology. 8th Ed. Philadelphia: Lippincott Williams & Wilkins, 2000. **B.** Courtesy of Dr. S. Shaw, Department of Surgery, University of Virginia. **C.** Courtesy of Dr. S. Lacey, Department of Surgery, University of North Carolina. **D,E,G,I.** From Fenoglio-Preiser CM, Lantz P, Listrom M. Gastrointestinal Pathology: An Atlas and Text. 2nd Ed. Philadelphia: Lippincott Williams & Wilkins, 1999. **F,H.** From Yamada T, Alpers D, Laine L, et al., eds. Textbook of Gastroenterology, vol 1, 3rd Ed. Philadelphia: Lippincott Williams & Wilkins, 1999.

Figure 7-7: A, photo. From Sternberg SS. Histology for Pathologists. 2nd Ed. Baltimore: Williams & Wilkins, 1997:554. **B.** From T, Alpers D, Laine L, et al., eds. Textbook of Gastroenterology, vol 1, 3rd Ed. Philadelphia: Lippincott Williams & Wilkins, 1999.

Figure 8-1: A,B,D–F. From Dudek RW, Fix JD. Board Review Series: Embryology. 3rd Ed. Philadelphia: Lippincott Williams & Wilkins, 2005:139. **C.** From Johnson KE. NMS Human Developmental Anatomy. Baltimore: Williams & Wilkins, 1988:269.

Figure 8-2A: From Johnson KE. NMS Human Developmental Anatomy. Baltimore: Williams & Wilkins, 1988:269.

Figure 8-3: A,J. From Sternberg SS. Histology for Pathologists. 2nd Ed. Baltimore: Williams & Wilkins, 1997. **B,D,E,G.** From Kirks DR, Griscom NT. Practical Pediatric Imaging. 3rd Ed. Baltimore: Williams & Wilkins, 1997. **C.** From Rubin E, Farber JL. Pathology. 3rd Ed. Philadelphia: Lippincott Williams & Wilkins, 1999:865. **F.** From Avery GB. Neonatology: Pathophysiology and Management of the Newborn. 5th Ed. Philadelphia: Lippincott Williams & Wilkins, 1999:979. **H.** From McMillan JA, DeAngelis CD, Feigin RD, et al., eds. Oski's Pediatrics: Principles and Practice. 3rd Ed. Philadelphia: Lippincott Williams & Wilkins, 1999:1579. **L.** From Eisenberg RL. Clinical Imaging. 4th Ed. Philadelphia: Lippincott Williams & Wilkins, 2003:301.

Figure 8-4: B(1),C(2). From Sternberg SS. Diagnostic Surgical Pathology, vol 1, 3rd Ed. Philadelphia: Lippincott Williams & Wilkins, 1999. **C(1).** From Rubin E, Farber JL: Pathology. 3rd Ed. Philadelphia: Lippincott Williams & Wilkins, 1999:1197.

Figure 9-1: A–C. Adapted from Shakzkes DR, Haller JO, Velcek FT. Imaging of uterovaginal anomalies in the pediatric population. Urol Radiol 1991;13:58. **D–F.** From Dudek RW, Fix JD. Board Review Series: Embryology. 3rd Ed. Philadelphia: Lippincott Williams & Wilkins, 2005:151. **G.** From Janovski NA. Ovarian tumors. In: Friedman EA, ed. Major Problems in Obstetrics and Gynecology, vol. 4. Philadelphia: WB Saunders, 1973:191.

Figure 9-2: A,B. From Dudek RW, Fix JD: Board Review Series: Embryology. 3rd Ed. Philadelphia: Lippincott Williams & Wilkins, 2005:152. **C.** From Fletcher MA: Physical Diagnosis in Neonatology. Philadelphia: Lippincott-Raven, 1998:369. **D.** From Sternberg SS. Histology for Pathologists. 2nd Ed. Philadelphia: Lippincott Williams & Wilkins, 1999:852.

Figure 9-3: (1–3). From Spitzer IB, Rebar RW. Counselling for women with medical problems: ovary and reproductive organs. In: Hollingsworth D, Resnik R, eds. Medical Counselling Before Pregnancy. New York: Churchill Livingstone, 1988:213–248. Courtesy of Dr. A. Gerbie. **(4).** From Gidwani G, Falcone T, eds. Congenital Malformation of the Female Genital Tract. Philadelphia: Lippincott Williams & Wilkins, 1999:81. **(5).** From Moore KL, Dalley AF II. Clinically Oriented Anatomy. 4th Ed. Philadelphia: Lippincott Williams & Wilkins, 1999.

Figure 10-1: A–C. From Shakzkes DR, Haller JO, Velcek FT. Imaging of uterovaginal anomalies in the pediatric population. Urol Radiol 1991;13:58; Markham SM, Waterhouse TB. Structural anomalies of the reproductive tract. Curr Opin Obstet Gynecol 1992;4:867. **D,E.** From Dudek RW, Fix JD. Board Review Series: Embryology. 3rd Ed. Philadelphia: Lippincott Williams & Wilkins, 2005:160.

Figure 10-2: From Dudek RW, Fix JD: Board Review Series: Embryology. 3rd Ed. Philadelphia: Lippincott Williams & Wilkins, 2005:161.

Figure 10-3: A. From Sadler TW. Langman's Medical Embryology. 9th Ed. Philadelphia: Lippincott Williams & Wilkins, 2004:352; Courtesy of Dr. R. J. Gorlin, Department of Oral Pathology and Genetics, University of Minnesota. **B,E.** Courtesy of Dr. T. Ernesto Figueroa. **C.** From MacDonald MG, Mullett MD, Seshia MM, eds. Avery's Neonatology: Pathophysiology and Management of the Newborn, 6th Ed. Philadelphia: Lippincott Williams & Wilkins, 2005. **D.** From Fletcher MA: Physical Diagnosis in Neonatology. Philadelphia: Lippincott-Raven, 1998:378.

Figure 10-4: A. From Sadler TW. Langman's Medical Embryology. 9th Ed. Philadelphia: Lippincott Williams & Wilkins, 2004. **B.** From Beckmann CRB, Ling FW, Laube DW, et al. Obstetrics and Gynecology. 4th Ed. Philadelphia: Lippincott Williams & Wilkins, 2002. **C.** From Warkany J. Congenital Malformations: Notes and Comments. Chicago: Year Book Medical Publishers, 1971:337. **D.** From Jones HW, Scott WW. Hermaphroditism, Genital Anomalies and Related Endocrine Disorders. Baltimore: Williams & Wilkins, 1958.

Figure 11-1: A–C. From Dudek RW, Fix JD. Board Review Series: Embryology. 3rd Ed. Philadelphia: Lippincott Williams & Wilkins, 2005:119. **D–H, diagrams.** From Yamada T, Alpers DH, Laine L, et al., eds. Textbook of Gastroenterology, vol 1, 3rd Ed. Philadelphia: Lippincott Williams & Wilkins, 1999:1186. **D, radiograph.** From Kirks DR, Griscom NT. Practical Pediatric Imaging. 3rd Ed. Baltimore: Williams & Wilkins, 1997:845. **F, radiograph.** From Avery GB. Neonatology: Pathophysiology and Management of the Newborn. 5th Ed. Philadelphia: Lippincott Williams & Wilkins, 1999:1018.

Figure 11-2: A. From Rohen JW, Yokochi C, Lutjen-Drecoll E, et al. Color Atlas of Anatomy. 4th Ed. Philadelphia: Lippincott Williams & Wilkins, 1998:235. **B,C.** From Kirks DR, Griscom NT. Practical Pediatric Imaging. 3rd Ed. Baltimore: Williams & Wilkins, 1997.

Figure 11-3: A. From Dudek RW, Fix JD. Board Review Series: Embryology. 3rd Ed. Philadelphia: Lippincott Williams & Wilkins, 2005:124. **B.** From Kirks DR, Griscom NT. Practical Pediatric Imaging. 3rd Ed. Philadelphia: Lippincott Williams & Wilkins, 1997:695.

Figure 12-1: From Dudek RW, Fix JD. Board Review Series: Embryology. 3rd Ed. Philadelphia: Lippincott Williams & Wilkins, 2005.

Figure 12-2: From Dudek RW, Fix JD. Board Review Series: Embryology. 3rd Ed. Philadelphia: Lippincott Williams & Wilkins, 2005. **Insets in C.** From Johnson W. NMS Human Developmental Anatomy. Baltimore: Williams & Wilkins, 1988:307.

Figure 12-3: A. From McMillan JA, DeAngelis CD, Feigin RD, et al., eds. Oski's Pediatrics: Principles and Practice. 3rd Ed. Philadelphia: Lippincott Williams & Wilkins, 1999:394. **B.** From Kirks DR, Griscom NT.

Practical Pediatric Imaging. 3rd Ed. Baltimore: Williams & Wilkins, 1997:245. **C.** Courtesy of Dr. A. Shaw, Department of Surgery, University of Virginia. **E.** From Swischuk LE. Imaging of the Newborn, Infant and Young Child. 5th Ed. Philadelphia: Lippincott Williams & Wilkins, 2004:220. **F.** From Fletcher MA. Physical Diagnosis in Neonatology. Philadelphia: Lippincott-Raven, 1998:225. **G.** From Kirks DR, Griscom NT. Practical Pediatric Imaging. 3rd Ed. Baltimore: Williams & Wilkins, 1997:246. **H.** From Bickley LS, Szilagyi P. Bates' Guide to Physical Examination and History Taking. 8th Ed. Philadelphia: Lippincott Williams & Wilkins, 2003. **I.** From Sadler TW. Langman's Medical Embryology. 9th Ed. Philadelphia: Lippincott Williams & Wilkins, 2004:395; Courtesy of Dr. M. Edgerton, Department of Plastic Surgery, University of Virginia.

Figure 13-1: Modified from Truex RC, Carpenter MB. Human Neuroanatomy. Baltimore: Williams & Wilkins, 1969:91.

Figure 13-2: Modified from Johnson KE. NMS Human Developmental Anatomy. Baltimore: Williams & Wilkins, 1988:177.

Figure 13-3: **A.** From Sadler TW. Langman's Medical Embryology. 9th Ed. Philadelphia: Lippincott Williams & Wilkins, 2004:445. **B.** Modified from Sadler TW. Langman's Medical Embryology. 6th Ed. Baltimore: Williams & Wilkins, 1990:373.

Figure 13-4: **A,E.** From Sadler TW. Langman's Medical Embryology. 9th Ed. Philadelphia: Lippincott Williams & Wilkins, 2004. **B,D.** From Siegel MJ. Pediatric Sonography. 3rd Ed. Philadelphia: Lippincott Williams & Wilkins, 2001. **C.** From Fletcher MA. Physical Diagnosis in Neonatology. Philadelphia: Lippincott-Raven, 1998:391. **E.** Courtesy of Dr. M. J. Sellers, Division of Medical and Molecular Genetics, Guy's Hospital, London.

Figure 13-5: **A.** From Sadler TW. Langman's Medical Embryology. 9th Ed. Philadelphia: Lippincott Williams & Wilkins, 2004:468. **B.** From Fletcher MA. Physical Diagnosis in Neonatology. Philadelphia: Lippincott-Raven, 1998:200. **C,E.** From Swischuk LE. Imaging of the Newborn, Infant and Young Child. 5th Ed. Philadelphia: Lippincott Williams & Wilkins, 2004.

Figure 13-6: **A–D.** From Swischuk LE. Imaging of the Newborn, Infant and Young Child. 5th Ed. Philadelphia: Lippincott Williams & Wilkins, 2004. **E–G.** From Siegel MJ. Pediatric Sonography. 3rd Ed. Philadelphia: Lippincott Williams & Wilkins, 2001.

Figure 13-7: **A,C,D,F.** From Siegel MJ. Pediatric Sonography. 3rd Ed. Philadelphia: Lippincott Williams & Wilkins, 2001. **B,G.** From Swischuk LE. Imaging of the Newborn, Infant and Young Child. 5th Ed. Philadelphia: Lippincott Williams & Wilkins, 2004. **E.** From Rubin E, Farber JL. Pathology. 3rd Ed. Philadelphia: Lippincott Williams & Wilkins, 1999.

Figure 14-1: **A,B,D.** From Dudek RW, Fix JD. Board Review Series: Embryology. 3rd Ed. Philadelphia: Lippincott Williams & Wilkins, 2005:86. **C.** From Sadler TW. Langman's Medical Embryology. 9th Ed. Philadelphia: Lippincott Williams & Wilkins, 2004:406. **E.** From Rohen JW, Yokochi C, Lutjen-Drecoll E, et al. Color Atlas of Anatomy. 4th Ed. Philadelphia: Lippincott Williams & Wilkins, 1998:124.

Figure 14-2: **A–F.** From Fletcher MA. Physical Diagnosis in Neonatology. Philadelphia: Lippincott-Raven, 1998. **H, right; I.** From Kirks DR. Pediatric Imaging. 3rd Ed. Philadelphia: Lippincott Williams & Wilkins, 1998. **I, right.** From Sternberg SS. Diagnostic Surgical Pathology, vol 1, 3rd Ed. Philadelphia: Lippincott Williams & Wilkins, 1999:963. **J.** From Fletcher MA. Physical Diagnosis in Neonatology. Philadelphia: Lippincott-Raven, 1998:296.

Figure 15-1: From Dudek RW, Fix JD. Board Review Series: Embryology. 3rd Ed. Philadelphia: Lippincott Williams & Wilkins, 2005:84.

Figure 15-2: **A,B.** From Dudek RW, Fix JD. Board Review Series: Embryology. 3rd Ed. Philadelphia: Lippincott Williams & Wilkins, 2005:94. **C.** From Rohen JW, Yokochi C, Lutjen-Drecoll E, et al. Color Atlas of Anatomy. 4th Ed. Philadelphia: Lippincott Williams & Wilkins, 1998:130.

Figure 15-3: A. From Bergsma D. Birth Defects: Atlas and Compendium. Baltimore: Williams & Wilkins, 1973. **B–D.** From Tasman W, Jaeger E. The Wills Eye Hospital Atlas of Clinical Ophthalmology. 2nd Ed. Philadelphia: Lippincott Williams & Wilkins, 2001. **E.** From Sadler T. Langman's Medical Embryology. 9th Ed. Image bank. Philadelphia: Lippincott Williams of Wilkins, 2003. **F,G(1).** From Kirks DR, Griscom NT. Practical Pediatric Imaging. 3rd Ed. Baltimore: Williams & Wilkins, 1997. **G(2).** From Sternberg SS. Diagnostic Surgical Pathology, vol 1, 3rd Ed. Philadelphia: Lippincott Williams & Wilkins, 1999:993.

Figure 16-1: From Dudek RW, Fix JD. Board Review Series: Embryology. 3rd Ed. Philadelphia: Lippincott Williams & Wilkins, 2005:204.

Figure 16-2: A. From LifeART image copyright © 2004, Lippincott Williams & Wilkins. All rights reserved. **B,C.** From Crapo JD, Glassroth J, Karlinsky JB, and King TE, Jr. Baum's Textbook of Pulmonary Diseases. 7th Ed. Philadelphia: Lippincott Williams & Wilkins, 2004. **D.** From Avery GB. Neonatology: Pathophysiology and Management of the Newborn. 5th Ed. Philadelphia: Lippincott Williams & Wilkins, 1999:149. **E.** From Fenoglio-Preiser CM, Noffsinger AE, Stemmermann GE, et al. Gastrointestinal Pathology: An Atlas and Text. 2nd Ed. Philadelphia: Lippincott Williams & Wilkins, 1998:43.

Figure 17-1: A,F,G. Image provided by Stedman's. **B.** From Spitz JL. Genodermatoses. Baltimore: Williams & Wilkins, 1996:51. Courtesy of Department of Dermatology, Columbia University, New York, New York. **C.** From Spitz JL. Genodermatoses. Baltimore: Williams & Wilkins, 1996:59. Courtesy of Ingrid Winship MBChB, MD, Cape Town, South Africa. **D.** From Fletcher MA. Physical Diagnosis in Neonatology. Philadelphia: Lippincott-Raven, 1998:130. **E.** From Gold DH, Weingeist TA. Color Atlas of the Eye in Systemic Disease. Philadelphia: Lippincott Williams & Wilkins, 2001. **H.** From O'Doherty N. Atlas of the Newborn. Philadelphia: JB Lippincott, 1979. **I.** From Weber J, Kelley J. Health Assessment in Nursing. 2nd Ed. Philadelphia: Lippincott Williams & Wilkins, 2003. **J.** From Spitz JL. Genodermatoses. Baltimore: Williams & Wilkins, 1996:177. Courtesy of Gilles G. Lestringant MD, Abu Dhabi, United Arab Emirates. **K.** From Sternberg SS. Diagnostic Surgical Pathology, vol 1, 3rd Ed. Philadelphia: Lippincott Williams & Wilkins, 1999:24.

Figure 17-2: B. From Weber J, Kelley J. Health Assessment in Nursing. 2nd Ed. Philadelphia: Lippincott Williams & Wilkins, 2003. **C,E.** From Fletcher MA. Physical Diagnosis in Neonatology. Philadelphia: Lippincott-Raven, 1998. **D.** From Emans SJ, Laufer MR, Goldstein DP. Pediatric and Adolescent Gynecology. 4th Ed. Philadelphia: Lippincott Williams & Wilkins, 1998:593. Courtesy of George E. Gifford, MD, Children's Hospital, Boston MA.

Figure 17-3: From Dudek RW, Fix JD. Board Review Series: Embryology. 3rd Ed. Philadelphia: Lippincott Williams & Wilkins, 2005:173.

Figure 18-1: A. From Dudek RW, Fix JD. Board Review Series: Embryology. 3rd Ed. Philadelphia: Lippincott Williams & Wilkins, 2005:178. **C,D.** From Sadler TW. Langman's Medical Embryology. 8th Ed. Philadelphia: Lippincott Williams & Wilkins, 2000. **E,G–J.** From McMillan JA, DeAngelis CD, Feigin RD, et al., eds. Oski's Pediatrics: Principles and Practice. 3rd Ed. Philadelphia: Lippincott Williams & Wilkins, 1999. **F.** From Fletcher MA. Physical Diagnosis in Neonatology. Philadelphia: Lippincott-Raven, 1998:188.

Figure 18-2: A,C (inset),E,F,I,J (inset). From Dudek RW, Fix JD. Board Review Series: Embryology. 3rd Ed. Philadelphia: Lippincott Williams & Wilkins, 2005:180. **C,G.** From Esses SI. Textbook of Spinal Disorders. Baltimore: Williams & Wilkins, 1994. **D.** From Kirks DR, Griscom NT. Practical Pediatric Imaging. 3rd Ed. Baltimore: Williams & Wilkins, 1997:314. **H.** From Jinkins JR, Leite CD. Neurodiagnostic Imaging. Baltimore: Williams & Wilkins, 1997:69. **J.** Courtesy of Derek C. Harwood-Nash, MD, Toronto, Ontario, Canada. **K.** From McMillan JA, DeAngelis CD, Feigin RD, et al., eds. Oski's Pediatrics: Principles and Practice. 3rd Ed. Philadelphia: Lippincott Williams & Wilkins, 1999:2118.

Figure 18-3: A. From Sadler TW. Langman's Medical Embryology. 9th Ed. Philadelphia: Lippincott Williams & Wilkins, 2004:182. **B.** From Crapo JD, Glassroth J, Karlinsky JB, King TE, Jr. Baum's Textbook of Pulmonary Diseases. 7th Ed. Philadelphia: Lippincott Williams & Wilkins, 2004. **C.** From Gold DH, Weingeist TA. Color Atlas of the Eye in Systemic Disease. Philadelphia: Lippincott Williams & Wilkins, 2001. **D.** Image provided by Stedman's.

Figure 19-1: A. From Dudek RW, Fix JD. Board Review Series: Embryology. 3rd Ed. Philadelphia: Lippincott Williams & Wilkins, 2005:188. **B,C.** From Fletcher MA. Physical Diagnosis in Neonatology. Philadelphia: Lippincott-Raven, 1998. **D.** From Avery GB: Neonatology: Pathophysiology and Management of the Newborn. 5th Ed. Philadelphia: Lippincott Williams & Wilkins, 1999:1271. **E.** From Rubin E, Farber JL. Pathology. 3rd Ed. Philadelphia: Lippincott Williams & Wilkins, 1999.

Figure 21-1: From Dudek RW, Fix JD. Board Review Series: Embryology. 3rd Ed. Philadelphia: Lippincott Williams & Wilkins, 2005:215.

Figure 21-2: A. From Pillitteri A. Maternal and Child Health Nursing: Care of the Childrearing and Childbearing Family. 4th Ed. Philadelphia: Lippincott Williams & Wilkins, 2002. **B.** From Gold DH, Weingeist TA. Color Atlas of the Eye in Systemic Disease. Philadelphia: Lippincott Williams & Wilkins, 2001. **C.** From Sadler TW. Langman's Medical Embryology. 7th Ed. Baltimore: Williams & Wilkins, 1995:136. **D.** From Gold DH, Weingeist TA. Color Atlas of the Eye in Systemic Disease. Philadelphia: Lippincott Williams & Wilkins, 2001. **E.** From Bickley LS, Szilagyi P. Bates' Guide to Physical Examination and History Taking. 8th Ed. Philadelphia: Lippincott Williams & Wilkins, 2003. **F,G.** From Sadler TW. Langman's Medical Embryology. 9th Ed. Philadelphia: Lippincott Williams & Wilkins, 2004. **H.** From McKusick VA. Klinefelter and Turner's syndromes. J Chronic Dis 12:50, 1960. **I.** From Nettina, SM. The Lippincott Manual of Nursing Practice. 7th ed. Philadelphia: Lippincott Williams & Wilkins, 2001. **J.** From McMillan JA, DeAngelis CD, Feigin RD, et al., eds. Oski's Pediatrics: Principles and Practice. 3rd Ed. Philadelphia: Lippincott Williams & Wilkins, 1999:2231.

Figure 22-1: From McMillan JA, DeAngelis CD, Feigin RD, et al., eds. Oski's Pediatrics: Principles and Practice. 3rd Ed. Philadelphia: Lippincott Williams & Wilkins, 1999:2232–2233.

Figure 22-2: A,B (top),C. From Sadler TW. Langman's Medical Embryology. 9th Ed. Philadelphia: Lippincott Williams & Wilkins, 2004:17. Courtesy of Dr. R. J. Gorlin, Department of Oral Pathology and Genetics, University of Minnesota. **B (bottom).** From McMillan JA, DeAngelis CD, Feigin RD, et al., eds. Oski's Pediatrics: Principles and Practice. 3rd Ed. Philadelphia: Lippincott Williams & Wilkins, 1999:2242.

Figure 22-3: C,D (photos). From Mufti GJ, Flandrin G. An Atlas of Malignant Haematology. Baltimore: Williams & Wilkins, 1996:73, 179.

Figure 22-4: A. From McMillan JA, DeAngelis CD, Feigin RD, et al., eds. Oski's Pediatrics: Principles and Practice. 3rd Ed. Philadelphia: Lippincott Williams & Wilkins, 1999:2232.

Figure 23-1: From Dudek RW, Fix JD. Board Review Series: Embryology. 3rd Ed. Philadelphia: Lippincott Williams & Wilkins, 2005:231.

Index

References followed by an "f" indicate figures; those followed by a "t" denote tables.

C

Caffeine, 176
CAH. *See* Congenital adrenal hyperplasia (CAH)
CAIS. *See* Complete androgen insensitivity (CAIS)
Canal of Schlemm, 113f, 114f, 115
Canalicular period, in lung development, 82–83, 82t
Cancer, colorectal, hereditary nonpolyposis, 159
Capacitation, 4
Cardiac muscle, 141
Cardiovascular system, 28–38
  arterial system, development of, 35–36, 37t
  atrial septum, 29–30, 33f
  AV septum, 3, 34f
  heart tube
    formation of, 28
    primitive, dilatations of, 28, 28f
  IV septum, 31, 35f
  SP septum, 29, 32f
  venous system, development, 36, 37t
Cataract(s), congenital, 116, 117f
Cat-cry syndrome, 152
Cauda equina, 97
Caudal dysplasia (sirenomelia), 15, 17f
Caudal eminence, 97
Cecum, 46, 47f
Cell(s). *See specific types, e.g.,* Beta cells
Cementoblasts, 127, 129f
Central nervous system (CNS), 92. *See also* Nervous system
  congenital malformations of, 99–101, 102f–105f
Cephalic flexure, 95, 95f
Cervical flexure, 95, 95f
CF. *See* Cystic fibrosis (CF)
CHARGE association, 94
Chédiak-Higashi syndrome, 124
Chemical agents, 175–176
Chest, funnel, 136
Chlorambucil, 174
Chlordiazepoxide, 175
Chlorothiazide, 175
Cholesteatoma, congenital, 109, 110f
Chordee, 72, 75f
Chordoma, 15, 101
Choriocarcinoma, 13, 13f
  case study, 14
Chorionic villus(i), 19
Chorionic villus biopsy, 146
Choroid, 113f, 114f, 115
Choroid plexus cells, 96
Chromaffin cells, 61
Chromosomal abnormalities
  numerical, 148–151
    aneuploidy, 148–149, 148f
    Klinefelter syndrome, 149, 150f
    polyploidy, 148
    trisomy 13 (Patau syndrome), 148, 150f
    trisomy 18 (Edwards syndrome), 148, 150f
    trisomy 21 (Down syndrome), 148–149, 150f
    Turner syndrome, 149, 150f, 151
  structural, 152–162
    Angelman syndrome, 152, 160f
    ataxia-telangiectasia, 158

Bloom syndrome, 159, 162f
    breakages, 158–159
    cat-cry syndrome, 152, 159f
    cri-du-chat syndrome, 152, 159f
    deletions, 152, 159f
    DiGeorge syndrome, 152–153, 160f
    Fanconi anemia, 158, 162f
    fragile X syndrome, 154–155, 162f
    Friedreich ataxia, 155
    HNPCC, 159
    Huntington disease, 156
    inversions, 157
    isochromosomes, 157
    juvenile myoclonic epilepsy, 155–156
    Kennedy syndrome, 156
    Machado-Joseph disease, 157
    microdeletions, 152–153
    Miller-Dieker syndrome, 153, 160f
    myotonic dystrophy, 155
    Prader-Willi syndrome, 152, 159f, 160f
    spinocerebellar ataxia, 155–157
    translocations, 153–154, 161f
    unstable expanding repeat mutations, 154–157
    WAGR syndrome, 153
    Williams syndrome, 153
    Wolf-Hirschhorn syndrome, 152
    xeroderma pigmentosum, 158
Chromosome(s), in cells during gametogenesis, 1, 2f
Chronic myeloid leukemia, 154
Ciliary body, 112, 113f, 114f, 115t
Circulation, fetal, 25–26, 26f
CLE. *See* Congenital lobar emphysema (CLE)
Clear cell adenocarcinoma, of vagina, 5
Cleavage, 6
Cleft, sternal, 136
Cleft lip, 90
Cleft palate, 90
Cleft vertebra, 134f, 135
Clomiphene, 174
Clomiphene citrate, for anovulation, 4
CMV. *See* Cytomegalovirus (CMV)
CN. *See* Cranial nerve (CN)
CNS. *See* Central nervous system (CNS)
Coarctation
  postductal, 35–36
  preductal, 36
Cocaine, 176
Coccyx, 133, 134f
Cochlear duct, 107, 108f
Coelom, intraembryonic
  formation of, 119, 120f
  partitioning of, 119, 120f
Collecting system, development of, 54
Coloboma iridis, 116, 117f
Colon
  ascending, 46, 47f
  transverse, 46, 47f
Colonic aganglionosis, 49
Colorectal cancer, hereditary nonpolyposis, 159
Common atrium, 30, 33f
Common ventricle, 30, 35f
Complete androgen insensitivity (CAIS), 76f, 77
Congenital adrenal hyperplasia (CAH), 61, 74
Congenital brevicollis, 134f, 135

Congenital bronchogenic cysts, 81f, 82
Congenital cataracts, 116, 117f
Congenital cholesteatoma, 109, 110f
Congenital deafness, 109, 110f
Congenital diaphragmatic hernia, 83, 120, 121f
Congenital glaucoma, 116, 117f
Congenital hypothyroidism, 90
Congenital inguinal hernia, 74
Congenital lobar emphysema (CLE), 81–82, 81f
Congenital malformations
  of CNS, 99–101, 102f–105f. *See also specific disorder*
  of ear, 109, 110f
  of eye, 116, 117f
Congenital syphilis, 178f
Congenital torticollis, 141, 142f
Conjoined (Siamese) twins, 8f, 9
Connecting stalk, 23–24
Contraception
  hormonal, 4–5
  postcoital, 5
Contraceptives, oral, 4, 174
Cooley anemia, 25
Cor deltiloculare biventriculare, 30, 33f
Cor triloculare biatriatum, 30, 35f
Cornea, 113f, 114f, 115, 115t
Cranial nerve (CN) VII, spiral ganglion of, 107, 108f
Cranial nerve (CN) VIII, vestibular ganglion of, 107, 108f
Craniopharyngioma, 97, 98f
Craniosynostoses, 131–133, 132f
Cranium bifida, variations of, 99, 103f
c-Ret, 54
Cretinism, 90, 138
Cri-du-chat syndrome, 152, 159f
Crouzon syndrome, 131, 132f, 133
Cryptorchidism, 72, 75f
Curves, vertebral, 135
Cyclophosphamide, 174
Cyclopia, 116
Cyst(s)
  congenital bronchogenic, 81f, 82
  esophageal duplication, 40, 41f
  lingual, 90
  pharyngeal, 89f, 90
  thyroglossal duct, 90
  urachal, 59
Cystic duct, 43, 44f
Cystic fibrosis (CF), 163
Cytomegalovirus (CMV), 171
Cytotrophoblast, 6, 7f

D

Dandy-Walker syndrome, 100, 104f
Deafness, congenital, 109, 110f
Decidua basalis, 19, 20f
Decidua capsularis, 19, 20f
Decidua parietalis, 19, 20f
Defective dentin formation, 127
Defective enamel formation, 127
Definitive adult kidney, 54
Deletions, 152, 159f
Delta cells, 43
Dental lamina, 127, 129f
Dental papillae, 127, 129f
Dental pulp, 127, 129f
Dental sacs, 127, 129f